Dennen's _____

FORCEPS
DELIVERIES

Third Edition

ATTENDING, OBSTETRICS AND GYNECOLOGY: Waterbury Hospital, Waterbury, Connecticut; St. Mary's Hospital, Waterbury, Connecticut

CONSULTANT, OBSTETRICS AND GYNECOLOGY: Charlotte Hungerford Hospital, Torrington, Connecticut

ILLUSTRATIONS: The drawings were done by Mr. Alfred Fineberg, Medical Artist, Columbia University, New York

Dennen's
FORCEPS
DELIVERIES

Third Edition

Philip C. Dennen, M.D., D.A.B.O.G., F.A.C.O.G., F.A.C.S.
Assistant Clinical Professor
Yale University School of Medicine
New Haven, Connecticut

F. A. DAVIS COMPANY • Philadelphia

Printed in the United States of America

Last digit indicates print number: 10 9 8 7 6 5 4 3 2 1

NOTE: As new scientific information becomes available through basic and clinical research, recommended treatments and drug therapies undergo changes. The author(s) and publisher have done everything possible to make this book accurate, up-to-date, and in accord with accepted standards at the time of publication. However, the reader is advised always to check product information (package inserts) for changes and new information regarding dose and contraindications before administering any drug. Caution is especially urged when using new or infrequently ordered drugs.

Library of Congress Cataloging-in-Publication Data

Dennen, Edward Henry, 1896–
  Dennen's forceps deliveries.

  Rev. ed. of: Forceps deliveries / Edward Henry Dennen. 2nd ed. 1964.
  Bibliography: p.
  Includes index.
  1. Delivery (Obstetrics) 2. Obstetrical forceps.
I. Dennen, Philip C., 1925–   . II. Title.
III. Title: Forceps deliveries. [DNLM: 1. Delivery.
2. Obstetrical Forceps. WQ 425 D398f]
RG739.D4 1989   618.8′2   88-20272
ISBN 0-8036-2511-1

Foreword

For many reasons, some good, some very bad, the forceps operation has come close to extinction in this country over the past decade or two. This, in my opinion, is a highly undesirable development, and I was delighted to hear that the author and the publishers of this book are reacting to a virtual demand from the obstetricians that the older edition be updated. Happily, there is an increasing realization among obstetricians that the near abandonment of the forceps operation in recent years has not been advantageous to gravida or their fetuses.

The generation of obstetricians that I represent was trained to use forceps with great frequency, even *routinely*. We believed that the advantages of the obstetric forceps far outweighed the disadvantages and that their use could move us closer to our stated goals of a healthy mother and a well child. In my opinion, that idea remains sound, although experience has demanded that we balance the risks and advantages of forceps against the well-known shortcomings of abdominal surgery. Cesarean section is much safer than it was 30 to 40 years ago, but an abdominal delivery still carries a maternal risk of death several times greater than vaginal delivery. This fact is often forgotten today in favor of fetal health and survival. However, both the mother and the fetus-neonate must be considered in obstetrical decisions. In the face of higher maternal mortality from abdominal delivery, it seems reasonable to consider a forceps delivery as an alternative when a cesarean section is to be performed for "failure to progress." Much of the time, the use of forceps will be rejected out-right (pelvis is too small; station of the vertex is too high); but in a certain proportion of cases (the exact frequency being dependent on the skill of the operator as well as other factors), the forceps operation still appears desirable and preferable.

There is a serious need for a book that illustrates in an encyclopedic way the intricacies of obstetrical forceps usage. The present volume is an admirable fulfillment of that need and was written originally by an acknowledged authority on forceps delivery and was updated by his talented son, who, coincidentally, was a medical school friend of mine. The description of forceps techniques in the older edition could not be improved upon and is included intact from the earlier edition. The present author has updated the indications and contraindications of the forceps operation and has put in perspective the usefulness of forceps in an obstetric milieu quite unlike that of the prior generation. The result of their joint work is that *Forceps Deliveries* is authoritative and readable and is certain to become a new classic on a re-emerging and important area of obstetrics.

Kenneth R. Niswander, M.D.
Professor, Obstetrics and Gynecology
University of California at Davis
Davis, California

Preface

Forceps Deliveries had its origin in the *Manual of Forceps Deliveries*, privately published by Dr. Edward H. Dennen in 1947. The Manual was used by his residents and his students at the Cornell Medical College and the New York Polyclinic Postgraduate Medical School. The book, completed with illustrations, evolved and was published by F. A. Davis in 1955. A second edition of *Forceps Deliveries* followed in 1965. It has now been out of print for many years. Numerous requests for copies have been received from practicing physicians, residents, and program directors. I have been told that a few copies that did not disappear from hospital libraries are protected and (as in my hospital) copied by individuals for their use.

Although the obstetrical goals of a healthy mother and infant are unchanged since 1965, the means to that end have radically altered. The day of the 4 percent cesarean section rate is long gone, but so also is the day of the 50 per 1000 neonatal mortality rate. Technology, medicine in general, and society in particular have induced changes in obstetrical thinking and practice. Too frequently, operators with forceps ability are made aware, following a successful delivery, that in other institutions or in other hands a damaged infant could only have been avoided by abdominal delivery. This is the reason for this book.

Many parts of the book are virtually unchanged from the original version, and credit belongs to the senior Dr. Dennen. In particular, descriptions of technique have stood the tests of time and also the specific efforts of an inquisitive son who, in over 30 years of active clinical practice and teaching, was unable to find a better way to perform or describe them. Material considered obsolescent or in conflict with modern obstetrics has been deleted. The 1988 American College of Obstetricians and Gynecologists (A.C.O.G.) forceps classification is used as reference. Alterations and additions to the book reflect current obstetrical literature and are an effort to make *Forceps Deliveries* pertinent and useful to both student and clinician.

P.C.D.

Contents

Introduction

The history of the obstetrical forceps is long and often colorful. There is evidence of single or paired instruments in Sanskrit writings about 1500 BC. Egyptian, Greek, Roman, and Arabic writings picture or refer to forceps, although it is presumed that most were used for the extraction of a dead fetus. The credit for the invention of the precursor of modern instruments for use on the live infant goes to Peter Chamberlin (about 1600) of England. Gene Palfyn (1649–1730) of Ghent independently invented a paired "mains de fer." William Smellie, in 1745, described accurate application and rotation to occiput anterior rather than the previously practiced pelvic application with traction, regardless of position of the head. The addition of a pelvic curve to the forceps is ascribed to him and independently to André Levret (1747), who also developed the French lock. Etienne Tarnier (1877) initiated the axis traction concept with a new instrument. Inventions, modifications, reinventions, and variants have led to the description of over 700 obstetrical forceps. Most of these, although fascinating, are of greatest significance to the obstetrical historian.

For centuries, the concept of the instrument was that of an extricating tool usually used in desperation in a difficult last resort situation. Prior to the advent of antibiotics, intravenous fluids, blood transfusion, and safe anesthesia, delivery by the abdominal route carried horrendous maternal risk. Vaginal delivery was thus mandatory, contributing to the forceps' reputation as being associated with trauma and often tragedy.

1

Sir James Simpson designed a forceps in 1845 that was scientifically calculated to the appropriate cephalic and pelvic curvatures. He encouraged the use of the forceps because "the infantile mortality attended upon parturition increases in a ratio progressive with the increased duration of labor." Joseph DeLee modified that instrument and in 1920 presented his concept of the prophylactic forceps operation. He stated that the procedure protected the maternal tissues and the fetal brain. This theory has never been scientifically proven or disproven. Although Dr. DeLee was criticized by his colleagues for interfering with nature, the concept of elective forceps was increasingly popular with practicing obstetricians. Many authors in the 1930s and 1940s reported superior fetal results with low forceps and episiotomy when compared with spontaneous delivery. Many institutions reported forceps usage in over 50 percent of deliveries.

Factors were at work to slow, then reverse, the swing of the pendulum. Cesarean section techniques improved. The safety of that procedure with the availability of blood replacement and antibiotics made it a better alternative than a difficult forceps delivery. Other forceps indications were removed by the increasing use of oxytocin in the treatment of dysfunctional labor and improved methods of monitoring fetal status. Decreased use of general anesthesia with increased and improved conduction anesthesia techniques, while adding a few cases, subtracted more.

The difficulty with in vivo forceps training under conduction anesthesia situations is obvious. In addition, many obstetrical training programs have de-emphasized forceps training. A few no longer have personnel capable of teaching the skill and knowledge necessary for proper forceps procedures. The statement that we are training midwives and surgical technicians has been attributed to Dr. Eastman. Finally, influences from without, namely changes in consumer attitudes, have had their effect. The demand for "natural" delivery has cast a difficult burden on the believer in elective forceps. Even worse for the practitioner is the fear of litigation, when the word "forceps," particularly in association with "mid," is almost an invitation to legal action should a result be less than excellent.

The status of forceps in modern obstetrics is constantly under discussion within the specialty. Controversy is only proper in the effort for improvement of results. Unfortunately, some reported studies have been poorly controlled, although it is realized that prospective controlled studies of this nature are extremely difficult. Various studies have used different classifications and terminology that confused and obscured results. The 1988 American College of Obstetricians and Gynecologists (A.C.O.G.) forceps classification is expected to aid in this respect.

It is the firm belief of the author that an outlet (A.C.O.G. classification) forceps procedure with median episiotomy has been demonstrated to give fetal and maternal results that equal, if not exceed, those of the spontaneous vertex delivery. This assumes that the procedure is performed gently and thoughtfully by a reasonably skilled operator who observes appropriate precautions and technique. Poor results can be anticipated with unsupervised neophytes, when the operator's manual dexterity is below average, or in cases of injudicious use of the instruments. The simple low (A.C.O.G. classification) forceps procedure is believed to be in the same risk category as outlet forceps with safety for mother and child. There are occasions when a mid forceps procedure will be indicated. This will be discussed in the text.

Of prime importance, then, is the teaching of forceps delivery. Detailed instruction in the use of the various types of obstetrical forceps is difficult to obtain. The old adage, taught for years, "Learn how to use one type of forceps and use it well," has done much to retard the interest in other types despite their admitted advantages under certain conditions.

Designers of forceps and their satellites and students, who became teachers, taught only the use of their favorite type. Other types were ignored except to emphasize their disadvantages. The numerous types in general use show that there is no universal forceps. Many an operator has experienced the sense of relief and the thrill of success following the use of one type of forceps after failure with another type on the same case. There were reasons present why one pair of forceps succeeded after another had failed. These reasons represented the advantages of the former and the disadvantages of the latter.

With the advent of special types of forceps, more advantages appeared as well as more disadvantages. Also, different techniques of application and traction were required. A thorough knowledge of the advantages and disadvantages of the various types of forceps, and the techniques of their use, will eliminate many of the bad results following blind faith in one type, or the "trial-and-error" method.

The ultimate object of this book is to show that there is a choice of instrument in delivery with forceps, depending on the existing conditions; that one should choose the type of forceps that suits the case rather than try to make all cases fit one type of forceps. To help in accomplishing this objective, the various types of forceps are classified. Their style of construction is stated. The advantages and disadvantages of each are emphasized. A detailed description of the technique of the application and traction for all forceps in general use is given, with reasons for success or failure and pitfalls to be avoided. The eight positions in which the fetal occiput may lie at the time of operation are taken up in order. Forceps use in the management of abnormal vertex or breech presentations is described.

A classification of forceps operations according to the station of the head in the pelvis is given. This is based on the four major planes of the pelvis, each of which serves as a marker for the forceps operation performed at the corresponding level in the pelvis. The four-level classification is essential in order to divide the long distance between high and outlet. It corresponds closely to the A.C.O.G. classification.

To get the best results in a forceps operation, there are certain fundamental rules that must be strictly followed. First, it must be considered as a surgical procedure, and as such, it should be given the thought, attention, dignity, and respect accorded to any other branch of surgery. It should be done by a trained, coordinated team consisting of, in addition to the operator and assistant, appropriate anesthesia personnel, a circulating nurse, and someone trained in resuscitation and care of the neonate. To be short of help in an emergency—and one might develop at any time—is a dangerous and harrowing experience. Any operator does a better job, with less risk and less effort, if he or she has good assistance.

The delivery room should be fully equipped and set up, ready for immediate use at any time and conforming to the recommendations of the A.C.O.G. Manual of Standards. The best equipment for fetal monitoring, ultrasound imaging, and pH testing is advisable.

Finally, the obstetrician should be familiar with the advantages and disadvantages of the different types of forceps and the technique of their use. This permits him or her to choose the type that is best suited to the individual case and carry that case to a safe and successful conclusion.

ONE

Prerequisites for Forceps Deliveries

The indications for obstetrical forceps may be maternal or fetal. Maternal indications include maternal exhaustion, failure of labor to progress, or bleeding. In cardiac or pulmonary disease, a shortened second stage of labor may be indicated. Similarly, a history of spontaneous pneumothorax, detached retina, and so forth, would contraindicate bearing down.

Fetal indications include signs of distress, malposition (including the aftercoming head), or the low-birth-weight infant (but not including the very-low-birth-weight infant—below 1000 grams). In the past, 2 hours of the second stage of labor was considered a fetal indication. It has been shown that prolonged labor, in monitored fetuses, is not specifically associated with fetal depression or morbidity. Thus, one can be more relaxed concerning arbitrary time limits in the second stage. Cases should be individualized and evaluated to determine causes of labor disorder.

Elective or prophylactic forceps delivery, as advocated by DeLee, is considered to be both fetal and maternal in indication by those who are adherents of this concept.

The prerequisites for a forceps delivery are of vital importance and should be emphasized. They are as follows:

The head must be engaged.
The cervix should be fully dilated and retracted.
The exact position of the head should be determined.
The type of pelvis should be known.
Appropriate anesthesia should be in effect.
Adequate facilities and supportive elements should be available.
The operator should have knowledge of the instruments, their use, and the complications that can arise.

Engagement

An unengaged head is considered to be a contraindication for a forceps delivery in all cases. The risk to both mother and fetus makes it unwarranted to attempt such a procedure.

Engagement is determined by the passage of the biparietal diameter through the plane of the inlet. Generally, it is accomplished when the leading bony point of the skull has reached the ischial spines. The station of the head is marked and recorded as plus or minus centimeters of deviation below or above the ischial spines on palpation of the leading bony point.

Cervix

Full dilatation and retraction of the cervix must be present. Should a lip of unretracted cervix be caught between the toe of the instrument and the fetal head, marked obstruction to rotation or descent of the head will be encountered. Also, the risk of cervical laceration is great. There is no place in modern obstetrics for manual dilatation of the cervix with the head under instrumental traction or for cervical incisions.

Position

A correct diagnosis of the position of the head is necessary in order to get a correct application and proper traction with the forceps.

Most heads should be delivered in the occiput anterior (O.A.) position with an accurate application of the forceps. This reduces the effort necessary for delivery and lessens the risk of any injury. Heads not in the O.A. position are rotated to O.A. either manually or instrumentally. If the position is misdiagnosed, followed by an incorrect application of the forceps and improper traction, there is increased risk of injury. Not infrequently, the diagnosis of position is difficult to make. Continued practice and constant alertness are important factors in maintaining a high percentage of correct diagnoses. This problem may be simplified if attention is directed to the sutures rather than to the size and shape of a fontanelle. Fontanelles may often be distorted or obscured by molding or caput formation. Three sutures, the two lambdoidals joined by the sagittal, forming a letter "Y," indicate the posterior fontanelle. An inverted "Y" to the left is a left occiput posterior (L.O.P.); an oblique upright "Y" to the patient's right is a right occiput anterior (R.O.A.); and a horizontal "Y" to the patient's left is a left occiput transverse (L.O.T.) (Fig. 1–1). In case of doubt, the sagittal suture should be traced to its opposite end. Identification of the anterior fontanelle is more readily made, since it is the junction of four lines meeting in the form of a cross. These lines are the two halves of the coronal suture meeting the sagittal and the frontal sutures.

Occasionally, on tracing the sagittal suture throughout its length, it will be found to be curved like the letter "U," with its most dependent portion closer to the sacrum than the symphysis. Also, each fontanelle is in an anterior quadrant of the pelvis. This should be recognized as an anterior parietal presentation caused by anterior asynclitism (Fig. 1–2). Thus, what was originally thought to be an anterior position of the head because the posterior fontanelle was found in an anterior quadrant, now will be diagnosed as a transverse position, rather than left occiput anterior (L.O.A.). Less frequently, the opposite situation will be found. In posterior asynclitism (Fig. 1–3), the posterior parietal bone presents with the inverted "U" of the sagittal suture closer to the symphysis than the sacrum and its extremities dipping into the posterior quadrants. This is likewise a transverse position and is found usually in a flat pelvis with an unengaged head.

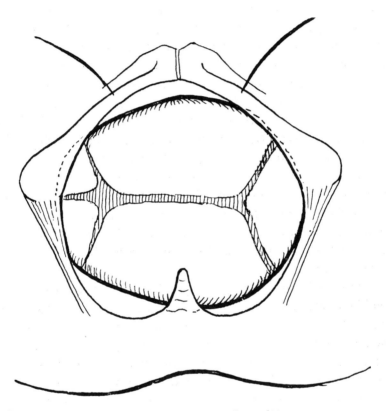

FIGURE 1–1. L.O.T. Normal synclitism.

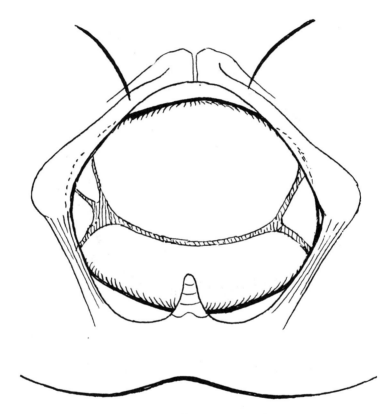

FIGURE 1–2. L.O.T. Anterior parietal presentation due to anterior asynclitism.

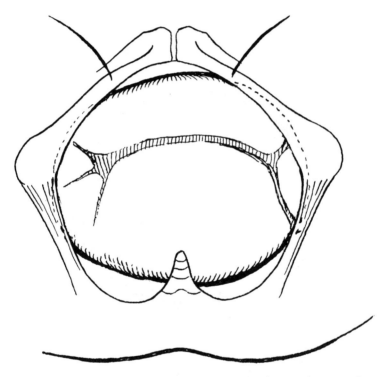

FIGURE 1–3. L.O.T. Posterior parietal presentation due to the posterior asynclitism.

If only one end of the sagittal suture can be felt and it is thought to terminate in the posterior fontanelle, a check may be made. By sweeping the examining fingers over the supposed occipital bone from one side of the "Y" to the other (the presumed two halves of the lambdoidal suture), another suture line, a continuation of the sagittal suture, may be felt dividing the intervening space. If so, it makes a fourth line leading to the same point and is, therefore, the frontal suture leading into the anterior fontanelle. If doubt still persists, the posterior ear may be palpated to establish the exact position of the occiput. However, this procedure is reserved as a last resort because of the risk of displacement and backward rotation of the head. This risk is less if the operator has a smaller hand. It has been said that a displaced head will come down again. Unfortunately, this does not always occur, at least, not in as favorable a position. Many of the technical difficulties of a forceps delivery may be avoided by not displacing the head. Occasionally, these difficulties are so great as to force the operator to abandon further attempts at delivery with forceps in favor of some other procedure originally considered unindicated or more hazardous.

Pelvic Evaluation

The importance of the clinical evaluation of the pelvis for adequacy in the fetopelvic relationship should not be underestimated. Routine antepartum and intrapartum pelvic evaluation is advised, but becomes particularly necessary should an arrest pattern develop. The obstetrician with a reasonable concept of pelvic architecture has a prognostic advantage in anticipating and avoiding certain pitfalls in practice. Pelvic contractures are associated with abnormalities of dilatation and descent, fetal malposition, dystocia labor, and, obviously, operative obstetrics. Cephalopelvic disproportion, a contraindication to forceps, must be ruled out. Forceps procedure indications change depending on pelvic type and relative disproportion.

Antepartum clinical estimation of fetal weight is a notoriously inaccurate art. However, it gains importance when pelvic evaluation indicates a potential inadequacy. Ultrasound evaluation of fetal size can aid in predicting a problem between a specific fetus and the pelvis that it must traverse.

The use of radiographic pelvimetry has greatly decreased over recent years. Although partially due to concern over radiation effects, there is also some lack of significance of the information gained with vertex presentations. The clinician can easily evaluate the outlet and mid pelvis for configuration and obstetrical import. The inlet and upper straits of the pelvis are naturally better evaluated with radiographic techniques, but this is frequently not necessary. Nonengagement of the biparietal diameter removes the inlet as a significant factor in that a contraindication to operative vaginal delivery would exist.

Simple illustrations of the significance of the pelvis are numerous. A post-trauma, fixed, anterior angulated coccyx may require fracture to remove obstruction to descent of the head. A history of childhood bony injury or back deformity can result in asymmetrical pelvic development and unusual diameters. Shortened anteroposterior diameters are associated with a higher incidence of shoulder dystocia, particularly with a prolonged second stage of labor and mid pelvic delivery. These and others demonstrate that pelvic evaluation is important in obstetric management.

Anesthesia

Appropriate anesthesia is indicated for any forceps procedure. This is particularly true if it is more than an outlet classification. Although reports have been published praising the safety and cost-effectiveness of a local anesthetic in the perineal body, this is felt to be far less than adequate for other than emergency situations. Minimum anesthesia is a good pudendal block. Many experienced operators find this procedure difficult and often inadequate. More preferable would be a conduction anesthesia such as low spinal or epidural. Under certain circumstances, a brief general anesthesia or even nitrous oxide analgesia may be effectively employed.

The association between regional anesthesia and the need for forceps delivery is well documented. Prolonged labor and a significant increase in malpositions have been reported. Anesthesia expertise, particularly the use of segmental blocking epidural techniques, appears to obviate the problem.

Facilities

As noted in the introduction, adequate facilities and support personnel must be present. Although the simplest forceps operations may be undertaken in a birthing room environment, the optimum conditions of a delivery room are usually advisable. In addition to the requirements as stated in the A.C.O.G. Manual of Standards, the operator should have at least level I ultrasound scanning available. In current obstetrical practice, the use of postpartum cord pH determination, particularly in other-than-routine forceps procedures, is advisable. This, of course, is in addition to careful antepartum fetal and maternal monitoring.

In a situation in which a forceps procedure (or cesarean section) is indicated for fetal status, the presence of a person skilled in newborn resuscitation and treatment is mandatory. The skill and acumen of the obstetrician can be negated by inadequate care of a previously depressed infant.

Instruments

A knowledge of the types of instruments with their advantages, disadvantages, technique, and potential complications is necessary for proper choice and use of obstetrical forceps.

The instruments may generally be divided into two types: classical and special. The classical type is composed of instruments that follow a style of construction and usage accepted as standard for years. The special type comprises more recently developed instruments that differ markedly from the classical in principles of construction and technique of use. Some instruments have special advantages under certain conditions; others are definitely contraindicated. Some fit the shape of molded heads; others round heads. With some, a more accurate application can be obtained with less manipulation. Others give a better line of traction.

The classical instrument consists of two blades each connected to a handle by a shank. The blade may be fenestrated, solid, or solid with an indented fenestration. It is connected to the shank at an angle that corresponds to the curve of the pelvis. Beside the pelvic curve, the blade has a lateral curve corresponding to that of the side of the fetal head, known as the cephalic curve. The tip of the blade is the toe, and the portion of the blade attached to the shank at the posterior lip of the fenestration is the heel. At or near the junction of the handle and the shank is the lock. Originally, forceps had no lock; but as the modern instrument passed through its various stages of development, there appeared fixed locks, semifixed locks, set screw locks, and cross bar locks. Almost all of the commonly available classical instruments in this country employ the English lock. Each blade contains a slot into which the shank of the opposite blade fits. In the French lock, one blade contains a pin that fits in a notch on the opposite blade.

CLASSICAL INSTRUMENTS

The type of *classical* instrument is determined mainly by its shank. There are two types of the classical instrument.

Elliot Type

The Elliot type forceps (Fig. 1–4) have *overlapping* shanks that impart a short, *rounder* cephalic curve to the blades. Due to the overlapping of the shanks, the blades must curve widely in order to attain a distance between them necessary to accommodate a fetal head with a biparietal diameter of about 9.5 cm. This bulging at the heels results in a more round cephalic curve, making the Elliot type forceps the instrument of choice for application to round, unmolded heads. The Elliot, the Bailey-Williamson, the Tucker-McLane, and its modification by Luikart, are examples of the Elliot type of classical forceps.

Simpson Type

The Simpson type forceps (see Fig. 1–4) have parallel *separated* shanks that result in a *long, tapering* cephalic curve. This type of cephalic curve makes the blade fit better on the longer, molded head. The Simpson, DeLee, DeWees, Good, Tarnier, Irving, Haig-Ferguson, and Hawks-Dennen forceps are examples of the Simpson type.

SPECIAL INSTRUMENTS

Special instrument types include a number of newer instruments that employ different mechanical concepts. They are designed to have certain advantages in differing clinical situations. The best known of these are the Kielland, the Barton, and the Piper forceps. These and other, more recent additions to the inventory of instruments are described and discussed in later chapters.

Complications

The complications associated with forceps use can be maternal and fetal. Maternal problems involve mainly soft tissue trauma including uterine, cervical, and vaginal lacerations, hematomas, bladder or urethral injuries, and episiotomy extensions. These have all been reported with spontaneous delivery. The frequency is greater with operative delivery, and the severity tends to vary inversely with the skill and judgment of the operator.

Related fetal injuries include transient facial forceps marks, bruising, lacerations, cephalhematomas, and facial nerve injuries. Less commonly, skull fracture and intracranial hemorrhage, poten-

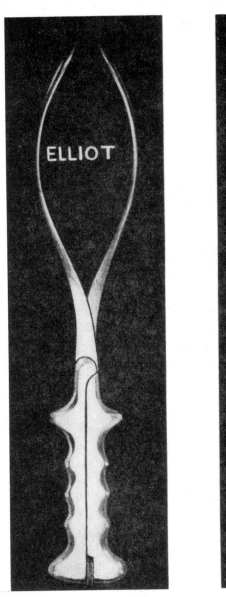
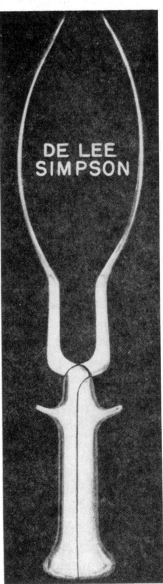

FIGURE 1–4. Elliot and DeLee-Simpson forceps.

tially with falx or tentorial laceration, are reported. Again, these injuries have been seen with spontaneous delivery, though in lower incidence, thus placing the onus on the operator. The more major problems generally indicate an injudicious use of the instrument.

The contribution of forceps to pediatric neurologic disorders is highly questionable. Cerebral palsy, mental retardation, and behavioral problems are believed to be more related to hypoxic episodes or other antepartum or intrapartum environmental factors than to operative obstetrics.

TWO

Forceps Classification According to Station of Head in Pelvis

Since early in this century, forceps categorization has been difficult, confused, and controversial. This partially has been due to problems with nomenclature and uncertainty in the application of terminology. The adjectives floating, unengaged, high, mid, low-mid, low, outlet, elective, and prophylactic have all been used to describe types of forceps deliveries. Each could have meant different things to different operators, although some terms were almost synonymous.

The American College of Obstetricians and Gynecologists (A.C.O.G.) issued their classification of outlet, mid, and high forceps in 1965. It was not universally accepted, probably due to the fact that the outlet category was unusually restrictive, while the mid category was too broad. It was unspoken, but generally accepted, that the majority of forceps deliveries were not outlet; therefore, by definition, they were mid forceps. This encouraged the use of the term "low" and possibly an element of intellectual dishonesty for the sake of the record. Many authors felt that mid should be subdivided in some way so that lower level procedures involving rotation, which have been associated with excellent results, would not be stigmatized.

In 1988, the A.C.O.G. released a new classification that is helpfully specific. It is quoted below:

Definitions

"1. *Station:* The relationship of the estimated distance, in centimeters, between the leading bony portion of the fetal head and the level of the maternal ischial spines. In classifying midforceps procedures, the level of engagement of the fetal head must be stated as precisely as possible. Engagement of the vertex occurs when the biparietal diameter has passed through the pelvic inlet and is clinically diagnosed when the leading bony portion of the fetal head is at or below the level of the ischial spines (station 0 or more).

2. *Outlet forceps:* The application of forceps when a) the scalp is visible at the introitus without separating the labia, b) the fetal skull has reached the pelvic floor, c) the sagittal suture is in the anterior-posterior diameter or in the right or left occiput anterior or posterior position, and d) the fetal head is at or on the perineum. According to this definition, rotation cannot exceed 45°. There is no difference in perinatal outcome when deliveries involving the use of outlet forceps are compared with similar spontaneous deliveries, and there are no data to support the concept that rotating the head on the pelvic floor 45° or less increases morbidity. Forceps delivery under these conditions may be desirable to shorten the second stage of labor.

3. *Low forceps:* The application of forceps when the leading point of the skull is at station +2 or more. Low forceps have two subdivisions: a) rotation 45° or less (eg, left occipitoanterior to occiput anterior, left occipitoposterior to occiput posterior), and b) rotation more than 45°.

4. *Midforceps:* The application of forceps when the head is engaged but the leading point of the skull is above station +2. Under very unusual circumstances, such as the sudden onset of severe fetal or maternal compromise, application of forceps above station +2 may be attempted while simultaneously initiating preparations for a cesarean delivery in the event the forceps maneuver is unsuccessful. Under no circumstances, however, should forceps be applied to an unengaged presenting part or when the cervix is not completely dilated."*

---

* From ACOG Committee Opinion. Committee on Obstetrics: Maternal and Fetal Medicine. Number 59, Obstetric Forceps. American College of Obstetricians and Gynecologists, Washington, DC, 1988.

This is essentially a four-level classification. The A.C.O.G. definitions cover only the categories for which there can be a valid or, as with mid forceps, a potential use in modern obstetrics. It is obvious that when the leading bony point is at the inlet, a higher category than mid forceps is inferred, although it is not an acceptable procedure.

The classification is a marked improvement. We must take issue, however, with the inclusion of the occiput posterior or oblique posterior positions in the outlet category when delivered as a posterior. This procedure has been demonstrated to require greater traction force, with the direction of force being critical to what, at best, is a more traumatic delivery than an occiput anterior.

In 1952, E.H. Dennen proposed a classification that related the station of the head (the biparietal diameter) to the four major obstetrical planes of the pelvis (Fig. 2–1). The planes are as follows: The plane of the inlet is bounded by the sacral promontory and the upper, inner border of the symphysis. The plane of greatest pelvic dimensions extends between the middle of the inner border of the symphysis and the junction of the fused second and third sacral vertebrae, having crossed the obturator foramen. The plane of least pelvic dimensions is bounded anteroposteriorly by the lower, inner border of the symphysis and the sacrococcygeal joint and laterally by the ischial spines. The plane of the outlet, quadrilateral in shape, is bounded by the sacrococcygeal joint posteriorly, the ischial tuberosities laterally, and the inferior border of the symphysis anteriorly.

When the effective diameter of the head (the biparietal diameter) is located at each of the four obstetrical planes of the pelvis, four distinct stations are established. (As one can see in Figure 2–2, the mid, low, and outlet categories are compatible with the A.C.O.G. classification.) The station of the head at forceps application determines the category, as follows:

High forceps delivery: Biparietal diameter is in plane of inlet; leading bony point is at or just above ischial spines.

Mid forceps delivery: Biparietal diameter is in plane of greatest pelvic dimension; leading bony point is at spines or below, to +2 station; the hollow of the sacrum is not filled.

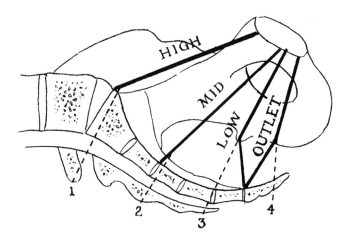

1. Plane of Inlet
2. Plane of greatest pelvic dimensions
3. Plane of least pelvic dimensions
4. Plane of Outlet

FIGURE 2–1. Four major planes of the pelvis.

Low forceps delivery: Biparietal diameter is in plane of least pelvic dimension; leading bony point is below $+2$ station; hollow of the sacrum is filled.

Outlet forceps delivery: Biparietal diameter is in plane of outlet; leading bony point is $+4$ station or lower.

This classification fits most cases. There are some exceptions in which the level of the biparietal diameter may be higher in relationship to the leading bony point of the head. These are cases that involve a larger infant, extreme molding, extension, asynclitism, or certain pelvic deformities. Unless these variable factors are taken into consideration, errors in diagnosis of station may occur.

The larger infant will obviously have a longer distance between the leading bony point and the biparietal diameter than will the smaller head of an infant weighing a kilogram less. There is also a greater tendency to molding with the larger head. Extreme molding lengthens the long axis of the head. Hence, the biparietal diameter is at a correspondingly greater distance from the leading point (Fig. 2–3). The estimation of this distance is of the greatest importance, since the biparietal diameter is the widest diameter of the fetal head that must pass through the maternal pelvis, and its level designates the true station of the head. With marked molding, in cases with the leading point on the perineum, the biparietal diameter may be at or above the ischial spines. What is often thought to be an easy outlet forceps delivery is later proved to be a difficult delivery of a head at low, or even mid, station.

Faulty attitudes such as varying degrees of extension of the head, including the extremes of brow and face presentation, and the abnormal attitude of asynclitism, influence the level of the biparietal diameter with relation to the leading point.

In extensions of the head, the biparietal diameter is farther from the leading point than in normal occipital presentations (Fig. 2–4). The greater the extension, the more the variation. In asynclitism, either the anterior or the posterior parietal bone is presenting (Fig. 2–5). Therefore, one extremity of the biparietal is considerably lower than the other. The actual station of the head depends on the level of the "pivot point," which is the midpoint of the biparietal diameter. The location of this point must be judged by the degree of asyn-

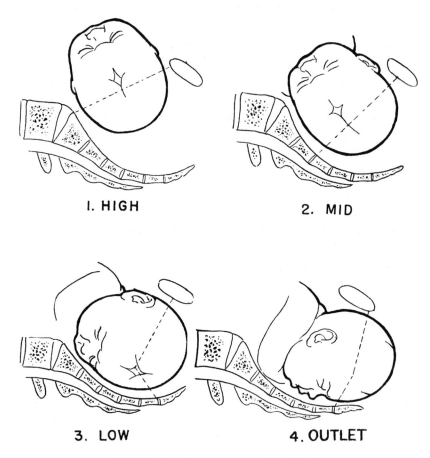

FIGURE 2–2. Four stations of the head.

clitism and the level of the leading point. The more asynclitic the head, the more one is apt to consider the head at a lower level than is the case.

Clinically, this is more frequent in anterior asynclitism with the anterior parietal bone well under the symphysis and the hollow of the sacrum being empty. The degree of asynclitism can best be determined by the shape and location of the sagittal suture. The greater the asynclitism, the more the shape of the sagittal suture changes from a straight line toward the shape of the letter "U." With the anterior parietal bone presenting, the "U" is upright. In a posterior parietal bone presentation, or posterior asynclitism, the "U" is inverted.

Deformities of the pelvis may predispose to and accentuate molding, extensions, and asynclitism. These deformities may involve any of the major planes of the pelvis and, consequently, affect the accuracy of the diagnosis of station.

At the inlet, molding is common in small gynecoid and android pelves, especially with posterior positions of the occiput. Asynclitism and extensions, even to the degree of face presentation, are frequently found in platypelloid pelves. With the head arrested at this level, the common mistake is to consider the head engaged when, in reality, the biparietal diameter is above the inlet.

Deformities of the plane of greatest pelvic dimensions, or midplane, carry with them similar factors as those of the inlet, and effect molding, extensions, and asynclitism. A transverse contraction in the anthropoid and android types frequently leads to a posterior position with more than average molding. A contracted anteroposterior diameter, due to a straight sacrum or a forward jutting sacral vertebra, leads to extension and asynclitism. Hence, most of these cases should be classed as high instead of mid, as the biparietal diameter is usually at the inlet. This knowledge should influence the operator to avoid the dangerous higher station procedures.

In the plane of least pelvic dimensions, the plane of the ischial spines, the greatest percentage of dystocias is encountered. The type of pelvis that carries the most difficulty at this level is the android. Here the molding is accentuated. It may be so extreme as to have the leading point touching the perineum when the biparietal diameter is

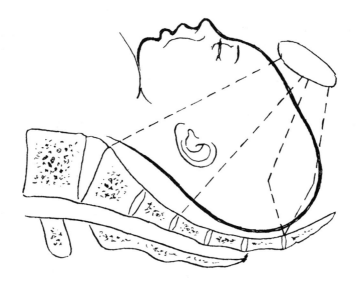

EXTREME MOLDING
MID O.P.

FIGURE 2–3.

still above the ischial spines. The common error in diagnosis in such cases is to label the operation low forceps rather than mid.

Deformity of the plane of the outlet, particularly with a funnel pelvis, predisposes to posterior positions and excessive molding. Here again, if the diagnosis of station is made by the leading bony point alone, the delivery will be classed lower than the actual classification.

Determination of the exact level of the biparietal diameter may be difficult to make. It is important that the phrase "at the spines" is correctly understood. When a leading bony point is at the spines, it has reached a plane that includes the ischial spines laterally and the sacrococcygeal junction posteriorly. In such a situation, the hollow of the sacrum is nearly filled by the head. The common error is to feel the fetal head in the anterior part of the pelvis, and to consider the vertex at the spines without investigating further to see whether the hollow of the sacrum is empty. The difference may be between a head that is in mid pelvis and one that is high or unengaged. On occasion, with complicated cases, an erect lateral x-ray study can be a valuable diagnostic tool. The exact level of the biparietal diameter can be determined, and it may show a previously unrecognized deformity of the sacrum to be the cause of dystocia.

In the average case, it can be assumed that the biparietal diameter is located at a certain level, depending on the level of the leading bony point, as has been indicated. In cases with extreme molding, abnormal attitudes, and in deformed pelves predisposing to those conditions, the biparietal diameter automatically should be placed at least at the next higher plane.

Visual evidence of the fetal scalp at the perineum does not necessarily mean an easy outlet forceps delivery. Without a systematized classification, there is a great void between the outlet forceps, in which the head is visible, and the mid forceps, which may be anything from the easiest procedure to a complicated delivery of a head at the inlet. This is one reason why the true mid forceps operation has fallen into discredit.

Many studies have been published concerning the results of operative vaginal deliveries. The terms "outlet" and "low" have been used interchangeably in many instances. Despite the problems of nomenclature, operator bias, varying skill levels, differing indica-

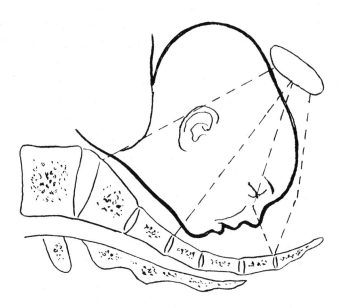

HIGH POST. CHIN

FIGURE 2–4.

tions, presence of monitoring, length of follow-up, and so forth, some general agreement has been reached. The outlet, or low forceps, procedure was considered preferable to spontaneous delivery by early investigators. The National Institute of Neurologic Diseases and Stroke Collaborative Perinatal Project tended to agree with the earlier studies. This large cohort, prospective controlled study measured many parameters, with a 4-year follow-up. Later studies agree with the safety of the low (or outlet) forceps procedure. Several, in fact, again suggest results superior to those of spontaneous delivery.

The case for mid forceps is more confusing. Data from the Collaborative Perinatal Project have been interpreted to support the opposing view of forceps protagonists and antagonists. The often quoted Friedman and associates analyzed the data and showed small, but statistically significant, adverse long-term effects following mid forceps delivery compared with spontaneous or low forceps delivery. Unfortunately, the risk factors (anesthesia, dystocia, distress) prompting the operative intervention were not documented, nor were mid forceps results compared with cesarean section results. In this study and others, it is patently unreasonable to compare the results of indicated mid forceps delivery to spontaneous delivery. Generally, the only possible alternative is cesarean section. When compared with abdominal delivery, the mid forceps operation appears to offer equal or superior fetal results, with the added advantage of much lower maternal morbidity.

The pronouncements of those who would abjure all mid forceps procedures should be viewed with guarded skepticism. There is a definite place for the anticipated easy mid forceps procedure. This presupposes a cautious operator who observes the prerequisites, uses appropriate technique, and employs the cognitive processes to avoid pitfalls and desist if problems develop.

Medical-Legal Aspects

There is considerable concern about the medical-legal aspects of forceps delivery in view of our litigious society. It is deplorable that well-trained obstetricians have stated that they will no longer use

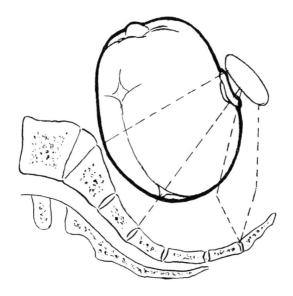

ANT. PARIETAL PRESENTATION
HIGH L.O.T.

FIGURE 2–5.

other than outlet forceps, fearing the potential legal consequences of a bad result delivered vaginally rather than abdominally. Thus, non-medical factors have been able to change medical management. Obstetrical education has been similarly affected in that a negative change has evolved in the teaching of this "mark of the obstetrician."

Equally deplorable is the tendency of the legal system to ascribe a damaged child to the procedure, or its performance, rather than to the circumstances that indicated the procedure. The malpractice suit is settled by "the preponderance of evidence." The operator must attempt to prove that the damage was incurred either prior to, or subsequent to, the procedure in question. This is obviously not easy, particularly in the emotion-charged situation of a defective child.

To paraphrase Dr. M. Rosen: Do good or bad obstetrics and get a good result, you don't get sued. Do good or bad obstetrics and get a bad result, you get sued; so you might as well do good obstetrics.

In consideration of the legal problem and, in fact, of good medical practice, it is important to document. The indications for the forceps procedure should be outlined to the patient and entered in the medical record. This discussion with the patient and/or relatives should be noted in the chart progress notes; it can simulate and indicate informed consent. The pertinent factors of predelivery and postdelivery fetal status, station, position, and attitude, the instrument and the type of forceps procedure, as well as the degree of difficulty should be recorded in a delivery note. The operator is also advised to make use of the laboratory facilities in unusual cases. Scalp pH readings in problem labors, cord pH at delivery, and pathologic examination of the placenta can offer potentially supporting evidence to the obstetrician, which is equally as important as the monitor record.

THREE

Technique of Application

Correct application of the forceps prior to traction is mandatory. All applications must be cephalic, that is, in relation to the fetal head rather than the maternal pelvis. The so called "pelvic application" has no place in modern obstetrics.

In a true cephalic application, the blades fit the head as evenly as possible. Thus, the place of application of the blade and the shape of the head must be considered. The blades should lie evenly against the side of the head, reaching to and beyond the malar eminences, symmetrically covering the space between the orbits and the ears (Figs. 3–1, 3–2). There should be no extra pressure at any one point. A correct application prevents injury to the head because the blades fit the head accurately and pressure is evenly distributed. The pressure is applied to the least vulnerable areas and is transmitted symmetrically to the normally symmetrical intracranial structures. Disruption of the falx cerebri or tentorium with intracranial hemorrhage is a risk when force is transmitted to an asymmetrical application such as a brow-mastoid application.

Correct application allows the operator to know the exact attitude of the head. Knowing the direction of the long axis of the head should ensure descent in the proper attitude of flexion, minimizing the force necessary and decreasing trauma to maternal or fetal structures.

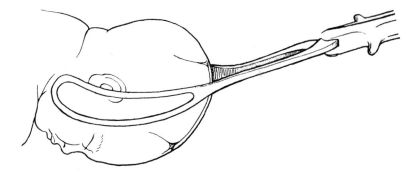

FIGURE 3–1. True cephalic (biparietal, bimalar) application.

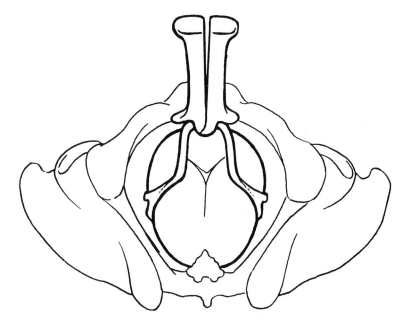

FIGURE 3–2. Correct application—according to the three checks.

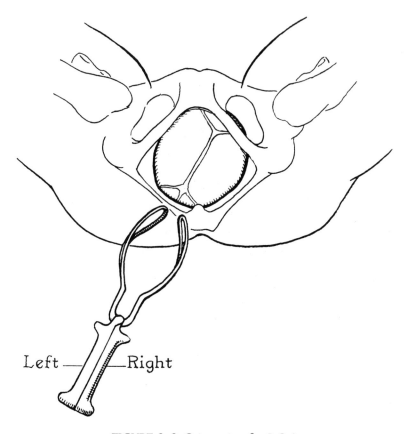

FIGURE 3–3. Orientation for L.O.A.

Technique of Application

The patient should be in the lithotomy position with appropriate prep and draping. As previously noted, with rare exception, adequate anesthesia should be in effect. The bladder should not be distended.

A vaginal examination is performed. If intact membranes are present, they are ruptured. Station, position, and attitude of the fetal head are determined. During the examination, station should be maintained if possible, since the higher the head, the more complicated the operation.

The blades are identified by holding them locked with the pelvic curve up, directed toward the patient in the position in which they will be when applied to the sides of the head (Fig. 3–3). The left hand of the operator automatically grasps the handle of the left blade, and the right hand grasps the handle of the right blade.

There are four cardinal points to remember when the occiput is in the anterior position. The *left* blade held in the *left* hand is inserted to the *left* side of the pelvis in front of the *left* ear of the fetus. The cardinal points shift to the right when dealing with the right blade. It is also important to remember that in all left-sided positions of the occiput, the left ear is posterior; in right-sided positions, the right ear is posterior. In posterior positions, the posterior ear is on the opposite side of the pelvis from that of the corresponding anterior position. That is, in a left occiput posterior (L.O.P.) position, the left, or posterior, ear is on the right side.

With the sagittal suture in the anteroposterior (A-P) diameter, the left blade is applied first. This facilitates locking the handles after application of the right blade since the lock is usually on the left. With the sagittal suture in an oblique diameter of the pelvis, the posterior blade (left blade for left occiput anterior [L.O.A.] and right for right occiput anterior [R.O.A.]) is applied first. By using the posterior blade technique, a splint is provided for the head, which tends to keep it in its anterior position and prevents its backward rotation to the transverse, or even posterior, position during the application of the anterior blade. This advantage far outweighs the slight disadvantage of the necessity of crossing the handles to accomplish locking in the R.O.A. position.

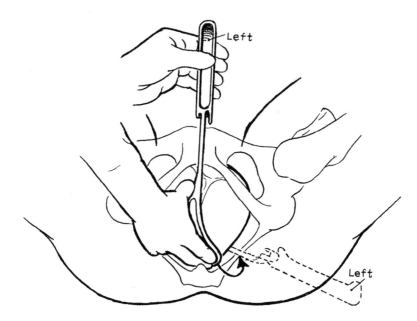

FIGURE 3–4. Introduction of left (posterior) blade for L.O.A.

Application for Left Occiput Anterior

In an L.O.A., the left ear is posterior. Therefore, the posterior blade is the left blade, the handle of which fits the operator's left hand, and it is introduced to the left side of the pelvis, in front of the left ear.

Temporarily, after discarding the right blade, the operator stands with his or her back toward the patient's right knee, holding the handle of the blade in his or her left hand by the pen grip. The pelvic curve of the blade is directed downward and the cephalic curve inward toward the vulva, with the plane of the shank perpendicular to the floor. This position directs the blade properly on its intended course along the curved plane of the head and the left posterior side of the pelvis to its intended place in front of the left ear. Any other position of the blade starts it in the wrong direction. The middle and index fingers of the right hand are then inserted into the vagina opposite the posterior, or left, parietal bone to guide the toe of the blade along the side of the head. The right thumb is placed against the heel of the blade, as the cephalic curve of the blade is laid against the curve of the skull. The force necessary to carry the blade into the vagina to its proper place is applied mainly with the thumb, rather than with the left hand at the handle. The left hand merely guides the handle downward over an arc, first outward toward the right thigh, then inward toward the midline, as the blade enters the vagina (Fig. 3–4). Force applied at the handle may be uncontrolled and unconsciously increased if resistance is met, thereby causing damage. The force exerted by the thumb at the heel is limited, and since it is applied directly on the blade is less likely to deflect it from its proper course. When the blade has been applied, if the pressure of the pelvis is not sufficient, an assistant holds it exactly as placed. In an L.O.A. position, the plane of the handle should be parallel to the left oblique diameter of the pelvis, at right angles to the sagittal suture, or approximately coinciding with a line connecting 10 and 4 on the dial of the clock.

The mistake often made by beginners is to change the handle so that it is parallel to the floor. This is an incorrect application unless the head has also rotated to the occiput anterior (O.A.) position with

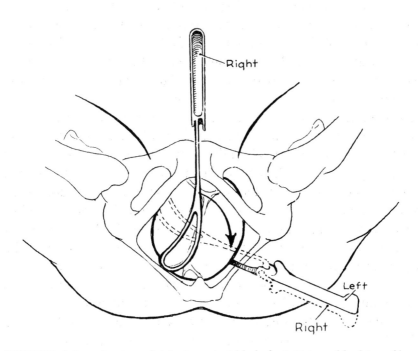

FIGURE 3–5. Introduction of right (anterior) blade for L.O.A. and locking of handles.

the sagittal suture perpendicular to the horizontal coinciding with a line connecting 12 and 6 on the dial of the clock.

In applying the second, or anterior, blade, the four cardinal points shift from left to right, and the operator changes position so that his or her back is now toward the patient's left knee. The right blade, held in the right hand, is applied similarly except that the toe is inserted anteriorly on the right side at a higher level so that it is adjacent to the anterior frontal bone. If inserted posteriorly as the left blade was, it has to be guided around the brow to the anterior, or right, ear by the middle and index fingers, which have replaced the thumb at the heel of the blade. In doing this, the fenestration may catch on a corner of the brow, causing the head to rotate back to a left occiput transverse (L.O.T.) position. Thus, the good application of the first blade is lost. The result is often the undesirable brow-mastoid application. The arc described by the handle of the right blade is longer in its downward component to carry the toe into the anterior quadrant over the right malar eminence.

When the right blade is in place, the handles are locked (Fig. 3–5). The left is not moved; since it was applied first, it is more apt to be in the correct position. The right is adjusted to fit it. If the handles do not lock easily, or if they diverge widely when locked, the application is incorrect. Usually, this is due to incomplete rotation of the anterior blade beyond the brow on the cheek and a short application. This is overcome by lowering the handle after unlocking it and elevating the blade by exerting upward pressure on the heel of the right blade with the middle and index fingers of the left hand. This carries it farther up into the pelvis and around to the side of the head. If this maneuver is not successful, the forceps should be removed. The position of the head should be carefully checked, and if it is found to be the same, the application is repeated.

After the handles are locked satisfactorily, the application is checked. This is done in three ways:

First: The *posterior fontanelle* should be located midway between the sides of the blades and one finger's breadth above the plane of the shanks.

Second: The *sagittal suture* should be perpendicular to the plane of the shanks throughout its length.

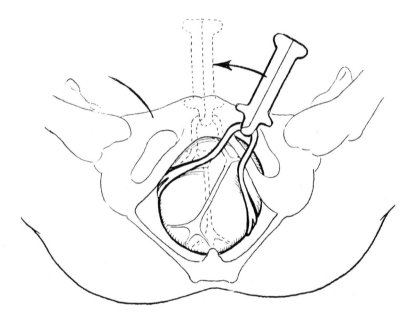

FIGURE 3–6. Rotation of L.O.A. with Simpson-type forceps to O.A. preliminary to traction.

Third: The *fenestrations* of the blades should barely be felt, if at all. Not more than the tip of a finger should be able to be inserted between them and the head. The amount of fenestration felt on each side should be equal.

Unless these conditions are fulfilled, the application is not a true cephalic or biparietal bimalar application. Readjustment of the blades is therefore necessary. This may be done without removing them. It is more easily accomplished after rotating the head counter-clockwise with the forceps, without traction, until the sagittal suture is in the O.A. position. Attempts at readjustment before rotation of the occiput to anterior often result in upward displacement of the head, backward rotation to L.O.T., and no improvement in the application (Fig. 3–6). Figure 3–2 shows correct application according to the three checks.

READJUSTMENT

If the posterior fontanelle is more than one finger's breadth above the plane of the shanks (first check of application), the correction is very easily made. The handles are unlocked and then elevated, one at a time, to the required level and then relocked. If traction is applied without this correction, the result is the same as traction on a de-flexed head. The pivot point of the head is above the center of the blades. Traction causes further extension of the head. This requires more force, with the accompanying risk of injury.

If the posterior fontanelle is less than a finger's breadth above or even below the plane of the shanks, the pivot point of the head is below the center of the blades. The application is in the overflexed attitude with the toes of the blades too far forward on the cheeks. Traction causes further flexion of the head. The correction is made by depressing or sinking the handles against the perineum one at a time, after unlocking them, until the shanks are at the desired level below the posterior fontanelle.

When the sagittal suture runs obliquely to the plane of the shanks (second check of application), it signifies a brow-mastoid application. Many of the milder degrees of this type of application

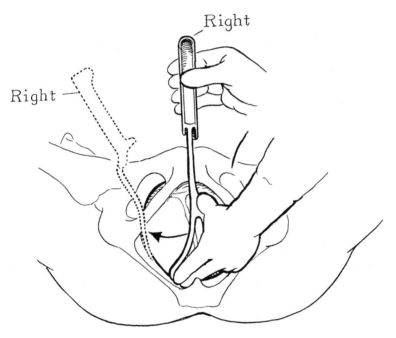

FIGURE 3-7. Introduction of right (posterior) blade for R.O.A.

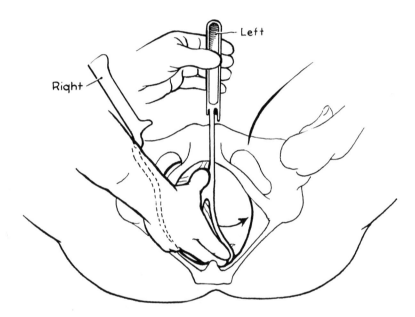

FIGURE 3–8. Introduction of left (anterior) blade for R.O.A.

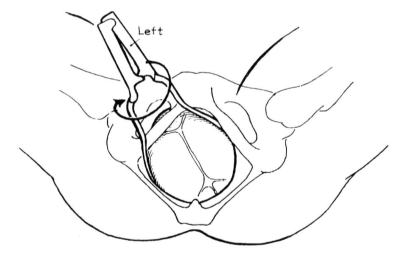

FIGURE 3–9. Crossing handles (left under right) for locking in R.O.A.

are not recognized unless the examining finger is passed along the entire length of the sagittal suture to determine its ultimate direction.

Correction is made by unlocking the handles and adjusting one blade at a time, usually the posterior one first, without removal. The handle is moved slightly away from the midline to move the toe of the blade away from the head. Pressure is then exerted on the heel of the blade with pressure in the opposite direction on the handle in order to shift the blade until the plane of the shank is perpendicular to the sagittal suture. The other blade is then adjusted in the same manner, although in the opposite direction, until its shank is also perpendicular to the sagittal suture. The handles are relocked and the position checked. Occasionally, the entire maneuver may have to be repeated if the result is not at first satisfactory.

If more than one-half inch of fenestration is felt below the head (third check of application), it signifies a short application. The toe of the blade is not anchored well beyond the malar eminence. This may cause the forceps to slip during traction. If the operator is not prepared, the blades may come entirely off the head, causing deep lacerations. In the correction, the unlocked blades, one at a time, are carried up farther into the pelvis until the fenestration cannot be felt below the head. The handles are then depressed and locked. After a final check of the application and anterior rotation, the next step is traction.

Application for Right Occiput Anterior

The technique of application for the R.O.A. is similar to that for the L.O.A. except that the order of applying the blades is reversed. The posterior blade in the R.O.A. position is the right blade and is applied first. It is held in the right hand and inserted posteriorly to the right side of the pelvis in front of the right ear (Fig. 3–7). Then the left blade, held in the left hand, is applied anteriorly to the left side of the pelvis in front of the left ear (Fig. 3–8). Since the standard lock is on the shank of the left blade, it will be necessary to separate the han-

Forceps Deliveries

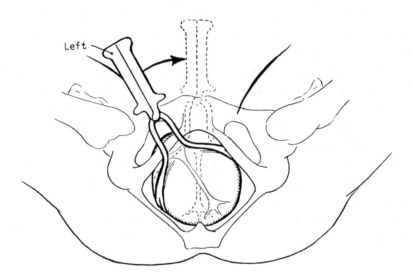

FIGURE 3–10. Rotation of R.O.A. with Simpson-type forceps to O.A. preliminary to traction.

dles and cross the upper, or left, handle under that of the lower, or right, handle in order to lock them (Fig. 3–9). After clockwise rotation to the O.A. position (Fig. 3–10), checking the application, and making the necessary readjustments, traction is begun.

FOUR

Traction

The ultimate and dominant function of the obstetrical forceps is traction in order to accomplish descent of the head in the birth canal. The only other primary function that we now consider is rotation in order to bring the head to the most favorable position for descent. In the past, forceps were used as levers under certain circumstances, to wedge the head into and through the pelvis. Since maternal structures served as the fulcrum, serious injury to mother and fetus was common. When destructive operations were performed, forceps were used as compressors, even perforators.

Compression is an effect, rather than a function of forceps, and great pains must be taken to minimize it. DeLee eloquently stated: "The accoucheur should always remember, when working with forceps, that he or she has a child's brain in the grasp of a powerful vise, and that only the greatest care and gentleness will save its wonderfully delicate structure from injury."

The student of forceps technique is impressed by compressive force when he or she places his or her fist between the toes of the instrument and squeezes the handles with the opposite hand. This often pictured (and used) technique employs the principles of a first class lever and applies compressive force to the skull. When one applies force at the finger guards, much closer to the fulcrum at the adjacent lock, very little compressive force is applied between the toes and the cephalic curve.

Strain gauge measurements of tractive and compressive forces to

53

the skull during forceps deliveries have been performed. The maximum compressive force is under 5 pounds with traction applied at the finger guards. This is considerably less than surmised by earlier authors. Compression is not directly proportional to tractive force and shows little change after application.

The negative compressive force applied by the divergent style instrument (Laufe) removes the forceps compression factor. Compression to maintain position of the instrument on the head during traction is still supplied, as with all instruments, by maternal structures, namely, the pelvic walls and intervening soft tissues.

Rotation of the head to occiput anterior (O.A.) is usually necessary prior to traction in the case of any position other than O.A. Depending on the pelvic configuration and capacity, rotation is usually easily performed with the biparietal diameter close to the plane of greatest pelvic dimensions. It can, of course, frequently be performed at a lower level.

If one thinks in the analogous terms of an egg in a tube, rotation is most readily accomplished with the long axis of the egg in the axis of the tube. An "off center" rotation results in friction and resistance. Similarly, the fetal head must rotate along its long axis, roughly perpendicular to the suboccipital-bregmatic plane.

When the forceps are correctly applied, a line connecting the toes of the instrument should meet the line representing the long axis of the head. Any rotation of the instrument should be performed with the toes describing as small an arc as possible, thus maintaining the long axis of the head in the same direction. Ideally, of course, that direction is perpendicular to the plane of the pelvis at the level of the biparietal diameter. Here the operator must think first in terms of the toes of the instrument and their movement. Secondarily, the operator must consider the effective widest transverse diameter of the head that must be moved: the biparietal diameter and its assumed level in the pelvis.

A most important consideration related to rotation of the head is the fact that classical forceps lose their pelvic curvature as they turn away from the anterior position. With a 90-degree rotation from O.A. to occiput transverse (O.T.), the pelvic curve becomes a lateral curve. The instrument no longer can correct for the direction of the birth canal. Consequently, the level of the handles must be lowered relative to the horizontal in an amount that increases with the degree of rotation away from O.A. Failure in this respect is reflected in difficulty with the procedure and will leave the telltale sign of increased marking of the anterior cheek of the infant.

Traction is divided into two elements, both of which must be considered: direction and amount.

Traction should always be in the axis of the pelvis. A picture of the pelvic curve as a stovepipe with an elbow at its lower end should be kept in mind when making traction. Force is applied in a plane perpendicular to the plane of the pelvis at which the head is stationed. Since the widest point of the head, the biparietal diameter, is being moved, it is the station of that point which must be considered. The higher the head, the lower from the horizontal is the line of traction. As the head descends, the line of traction moves forward in a curved line following the curve of the sacrum, then upward through the outlet. The pelvic curve of the classical instrument directs the handles in a plane obliquely anterior to the plane of the pelvis at which the head is stationed. Therefore, traction in the direction of the handles results in the force being wasted against the symphysis, with the possibility of accompanying injury and little or no advancement of the head (Fig. 4–1).

To apply the force in the plane of least resistance, that is, the axis of the pelvis, the axis traction principle must be employed. This may be accomplished manually. One hand grasps the shanks and the other hand the handles at the finger guards. Force is exerted in two directions: downward with the hand on the shanks, and outward with the hand on the handles. If the operator is standing, a downward push with the palm of the hand on the shanks results in the Pajot maneuver. For those whose preference is the seated position, the fingers of the hand on the shanks pull vertically downward in the Saxtorph maneuver (Fig. 4–2). The resultant force, or vector, is in a direction determined by the relative strengths of the outward and downward forces. This method is followed by varying degrees of success, depending on the skill of the operator and the station of the head. The higher the head, the more difficult it is to get axis traction by the manual method. Axis traction is best obtained with some

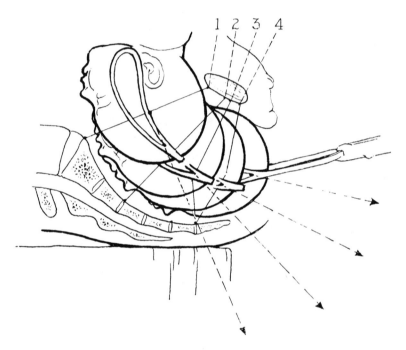

FIGURE 4–1. Showing line of axis traction (perpendicular to the plane of the pelvis at which the head is stationed) at different planes of the pelvis. (1) High. (2) Mid. (3) Low. (4) Outlet.

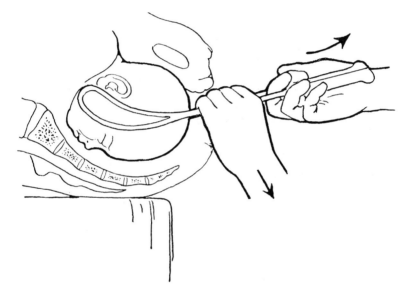

FIGURE 4-2. Manual method of axis traction—Pajot-Saxtorph maneuver.

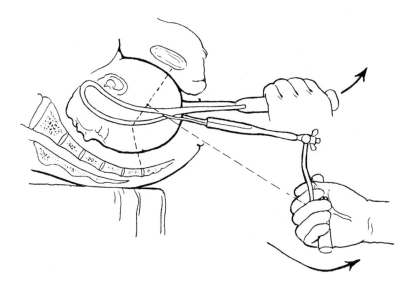

FIGURE 4–3. Instrumental axis traction. (1) Irving.

form of axis traction attachment, permitting traction to be applied in a lower plane, approaching that of the pelvic axis (Figs. 4–3, 4–4, 4–5, 4–6).

The amount of tractive force should be the least possible to accomplish the necessary descent. It is important that the operator remember that the procedure is not a contest of strength. Rather, it requires thought, skill, and finesse in following the planes of least resistance.

Studies have shown that the maximum pull along the proper axis should never exceed 45 pounds in a primipara and 30 pounds in a multipara. Most deliveries are accomplished with less force. Judging this amount of pull becomes relatively easy if one experiments with a traction measuring instrument or even orthopedic weights in a bag hung over a pulley. An experienced operator working with the manikin can supply appropriate countertraction to the efforts of the student.

As with the vectored traction direction, the amount of vectored force is difficult to deduce from muscle strength applied outward and downward on the instrument. This is the reason for the often advised use of an instrumental axis traction in other than the simplest cases. Although an axis traction forceps such as the DeWees may be used, the simpler use of the Bill axis traction handle on the finger guards can suffice. Similarly, special instruments with reverse pelvic curve or mechanically variable pelvic curve may be employed. In these instances, the vectored force becomes automatic for direction and amount when pull is applied to the handle. Another important consideration is that less total muscle power is required and the operator can appear more relaxed to nonmedical observers in the delivery suite.

Traction may be applied from either the sitting or the standing position, depending on the operator's preference. The seated position is felt by some to be preferable because of greater ease in gaining axis traction. The seat should be directly in front of the patient. It may be adjustable, but it must be stable. If standing, the operator adjusts position so that the dominant hand can be used for traction. Posture should be erect with the feet in a "fighter's stance" to maintain balance in case of sudden advancement or slippage of the forceps. Also, for control, the arms should never be extended. Rather, the elbows

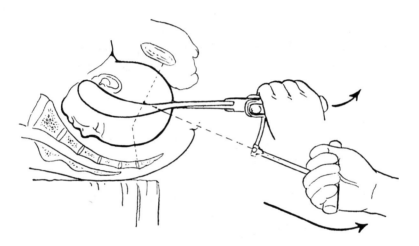

FIGURE 4–4. Instrumental axis traction. (2) Tucker-McLane, solid blades with Bill handle.

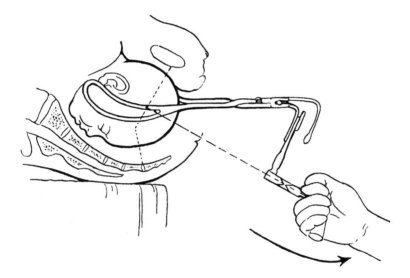

FIGURE 4–5. Instrumental axis traction. (3) DeWees.

Forceps Deliveries

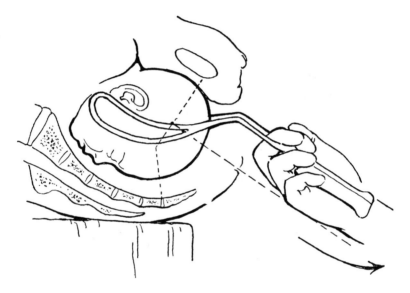

FIGURE 4–6. Instrumental axis traction. (4) Hawks-Dennen.

should be close to the sides, using shoulder and arm musculature instead of leaning backward using back and leg muscles. If the instrument has no axis traction attachment, the handles rest in the upturned palm of the dominant hand. The shanks separate the middle and index fingers that grasp the finger guards in the Elliot type of forceps. If a Simpson type is used, the middle finger occupies the space between the shanks, and the adjacent fingers grasp the finger guards. Compression of the fetal head from squeezing the handles is avoided.

The nondominant hand grasps the shanks close to the vulva. This is from below if sitting; from above if standing. This hand becomes the fulcrum hand for the Saxtorph or Pajot maneuvers, exerting downward pressure.

The traction hand applies traction outward in the direction of the handles, and the fulcrum hand pulls or pushes directly toward the floor. The result of these two forces tends toward axis traction. As the head distends the perineum and the occiput passes under the symphysis, the direction of the pull changes to follow a curved plane forward and upward. This change in direction is carried out gradually and only during traction, following the plane of least resistance. Observation of the relationship between the upper edge of the blade and the scalp adjacent to it can help in determining the direction of pull. The head tends to keep its long axis close to the axis of the pelvis, held by pressure from maternal structures. If the operator elevates the forceps too soon, the head cannot extend and the scalp appears to sink in relation to the upper edge of the blade. Conversely, late elevation of the instrument during traction results in the scalp rising as the head extends. The operator can then adjust the direction of pull accordingly.

Traction is made with a steady pull that is gradually increased in intensity, sustained for a definite interval, and then gradually relaxed. Under appropriate circumstances, and ideally, the timing should coincide with a uterine contraction and bearing down by the patient. The amount of force necessary for a gradual advance of the head and the number of tractions necessary for delivery vary with the case. Careful monitoring of the fetal heart should be maintained during rest periods between contractions. Monitoring equipment may quickly be removed when delivery is imminent.

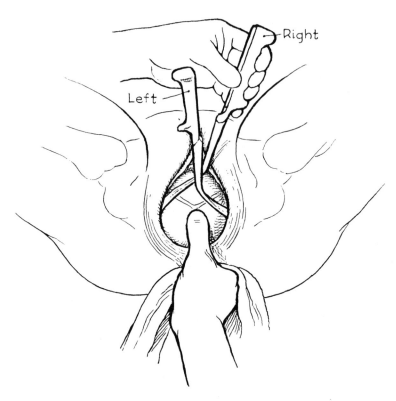

FIGURE 4–7. Removal of forceps while head is controlled by the modified Ritgen maneuver.

Performance of an episiotomy may be before traction or when the perineum is being distended by the head. Adherents of late episiotomy have the advantages of the rectum being pushed posteriorly out of the field and of less bleeding due to compression of the vessels in the distended perineum. Early episiotomy results in less traction force being needed. Early injury to soft parts in traction is avoided. The risk of a "buttonhole" rectal injury from the scissors can be prevented by the use of two spread fingers to depress the anterior rectum away from the incision site.

It is felt that if episiotomy is performed, it should be median except in rare circumstances: very unusual anatomy, previous fistula repair, or, possibly, Crohn's disease.

In extension of the head over the perineum, the handles are elevated by the fulcrum hand, leaving the traction hand free to perform a Ritgen maneuver. The handles should not be elevated higher than about 45 degrees above the horizontal, to protect against sulcus lacerations. At this time, the fingers, protected by a sterile towel, catch the chin through the perineum behind the anus, preventing the head from receding. The uncovered thumb of the same hand is placed directly against the occiput to prevent a precipitous advance of the head during the removal of the blades.

The blades are removed by a reversal of the motion used in applying them. The right blade is removed first. After unlocking, the handle of the right blade is carried over an arc toward the left groin and up to the symphysis. This is performed with the hand that is not occupied in the Ritgen maneuver. As the handle is elevated, it is rotated so that the blade emerges from the vagina across the occiput in a curved plane, with the cephalic curve of the blade following the curve of the head (Fig. 4–7). The left blade is removed with the same hand in a similar manner, toward the right side.

If resistance is encountered in removing the right blade, the left may be removed first. If both blades tend to stick, traction is not made on the handle because of the risk of injury to both the mother and the fetus from forcible extraction. If necessary due to resistance, it is acceptable to deliver the head with one or both blades in situ. After removal of the forceps, the head is delivered by the modified Ritgen maneuver. Restitution is completed manually. The shoulders and body are delivered in the usual manner.

FIVE

Transverse Positions of the Occiput

In the left occiput transverse (L.O.T.) position, it is often difficult to get a good application with the classical instrument. It is even more difficult in the right occiput transverse (R.O.T.) position because the handles must be crossed to lock them, and an accurate application may be lost by this maneuver. An alternative preferred by many obstetricians is the use of a special instrument (refer to later chapters). Before applying the blades, the operator may choose to rotate the head digitally or manually to the anterior position.

Digital and Manual Rotation

LEFT OCCIPUT TRANSVERSE

Digital rotation, which is occasionally successful, can make the more complicated manual rotation maneuver unnecessary. It may be used with or without anesthesia to supplement any rotational tendency evoked by the patient's bearing-down efforts. In digital rotation, the tips of the index and middle fingers of the right hand are placed in the anterior segment of the lambdoidal suture near the posterior fontanelle. The elevated edge of the anterior parietal bone offers re-

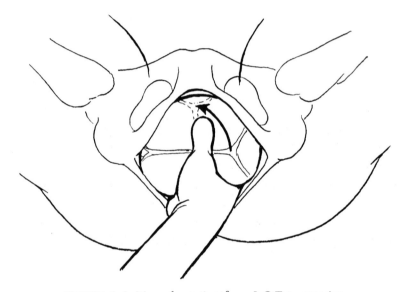

FIGURE 5–1. Manual rotation from L.O.T. to anterior.

sistance to the fingertips, so that when a lifting motion is carried out, the occiput may be turned in a counterclockwise direction to the left occiput anterior (L.O.A.) or even the occiput anterior (O.A.) position. The thumb may also be used with gentle downward pressure more anteriorly on the parietal bone to aid this rotation. Counterpressure with the fundal hand tends to fix the head in the new position. If delivery is appropriate at this time, the two rotating fingers are slipped behind the posterior parietal bone to prevent backward rotation and act as a guide to the introduction of the left (posterior) blade.

If digital rotation is unsuccessful, the manual maneuver is used. The hand used in the rotation depends on the position of the head. In left-sided positions, rotation is accomplished with the right hand, since that is the hand used later to guide the introduction of the posterior, or left, blade. The four fingers of the right hand are introduced into the vagina behind the posterior parietal bone with the palm up and the thumb over the anterior parietal bone. The head is grasped with the tips of the fingers and thumb. If the entire hand is introduced into the vagina, the head may be displaced or even disengaged. This should be avoided, since the higher the head, the harder and more dangerous will be the operation. The head is flexed and rotated in a counterclockwise direction to the anterior position, or at least to the oblique anterior (Fig. 5–1). Simultaneously, the left hand, placed on the abdomen, pulls the back of the child toward the midline. When this has been accomplished, pressure is placed on the fundus to fix the head in the new position. To prevent the head from rotating back to its original position, only the thumb of the right hand is removed from the vagina, leaving the four fingers in place to splint the head and guide the introduction of the left blade in the usual manner (Figs. 5–2, 5–3). After the left blade has been applied, an assistant holds the handle firmly, exerting a slight amount of force in the direction of the patient's left leg. This presses the toe of the blade against the fetal left cheek and keeps the head in the anterior position. The right blade is introduced in the usual manner. This blade must be introduced high above the posterior frontal eminence to avoid this obstruction. The handle is moved toward the patient's left thigh to shift the toe slightly away from the obstructing anterior frontal eminence. The blade is then lifted with the middle and index

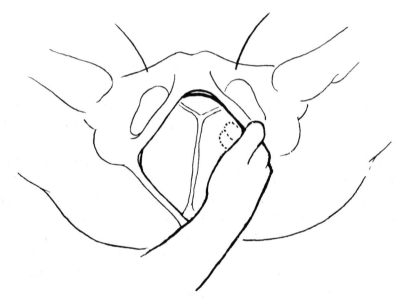

FIGURE 5-2. I.O.A. after manual rotation from L.O.T. Fingers of right hand in place, preventing backward rotation of the head. Thumb is removed in preparation for introduction of posterior, or left, blade.

fingers of the left hand, which have replaced the thumb at the heel, in order to bring it over the anterior parietal bone. If the fenestration catches on the frontal eminence, the head will rotate back to the L.O.T. position and the result may be a brow-mastoid application. After locking the shanks, the application is checked. If the head is in the L.O.A. position, rotation to the anteroposterior (O.A.) diameter is completed and the necessary readjustments are made before traction is begun. If the application is unsatisfactory after two attempts at readjustment, both blades are removed, the position is checked, and the procedure is repeated.

RIGHT OCCIPUT TRANSVERSE

In this position, the rotating and splinting hand is the left one. After rotation, the right, or posterior, blade is held in the right hand and inserted to the right side of the pelvis over the right ear. The left, or anterior, blade, held in the left hand, is introduced high on the left side of the pelvis opposite the left ear in a similar manner as was the anterior blade in the L.O.T. position. The handles must be crossed in order to lock them, since the lock is on the left shank. The head, if in the right occiput anterior (R.O.A.) position, is rotated without traction to the anteroposterior diameter, the application is checked, the necessary readjustments are made, and traction and delivery are carried out in the usual manner.

In general, the station of the head gives an indication for the choice of the digital or the manual maneuver to be tried. With the head close to the plane of the outlet, the digital maneuver is chosen since there is insufficient room for the manual maneuver without displacement of the head. With the head at slightly higher station, the digital maneuver is less likely to be successful, and there is room to try the manual maneuver without the necessity of the initial displacement of the head.

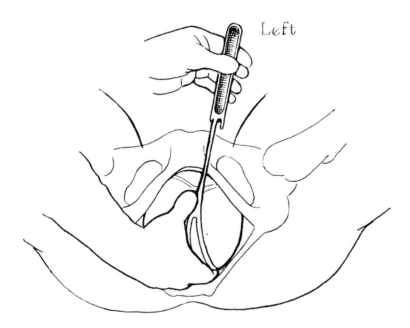

Left

FIGURE 5–3. Insertion of left blade (Simpson type) to L.O.A. after manual rotation from L.O.T.

Instrumental Rotation

LEFT OCCIPUT TRANSVERSE

An accurate application of forceps to the head in the transverse position is more difficult to accomplish than in the oblique position, because the anterior blade has to be carried, or "wandered," over a longer arc around the face to the anterior ear directly under the symphysis. In doing this, more points of obstruction may be met. When a proper application is accomplished, the plane of the shanks is directed toward the side on which the occiput lies, obliquely away from the midline of the long axis of the patient at an angle of about 50 degrees. The amount of deviation depends on the degree of the pelvic curve of the forceps and the position of the head. The plane of the shanks deviates from the horizontal depending on the level of the biparietal diameter since the instrumental pelvic curve is lost in a transverse application.

The wandering maneuver of applying the anterior blade to the transverse head is more easily accomplished with the Elliot type of forceps. Its rounder cephalic curve tends to offer less resistance than the Simpson while passing under the symphysis. Also, the overlapping shanks offer less resistance to rotation than the spread shanks of the Simpson-type instrument.

The left blade is introduced first, directly posteriorly instead of to the left side of the patient. Therefore, the approach differs from that of the anterior position in that the plane of the shank is not perpendicular to the horizontal, but runs obliquely to it, in order to allow for the pelvic curve of the blade. The toe of the blade is directly posterior and the blade parallels the plane of the sacrum with the shank following obliquely to the plane of the sacrum. The blade hugs the head to avoid obstruction. As the blade enters the vagina, the handle is lowered until it reaches a point just below the horizontal, following the plane of least resistance. The fenestration should barely be felt below the head. The angle the handle makes with the horizontal will depend on the station of the head. "The higher the head, the lower the handle" (Fig. 5–4).

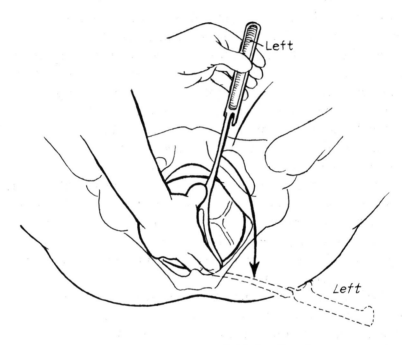

FIGURE 5–4. Introduction of posterior, or left, blade (Elliot) for instrumental rotation of L.O.T. to O.A.

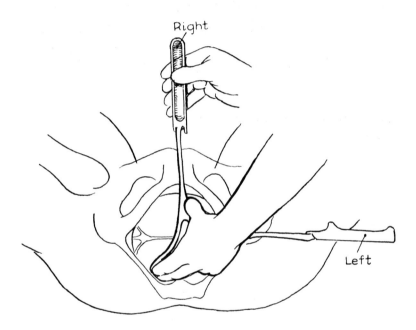

FIGURE 5–5. Introduction of anterior, or right, blade (Elliot) for instrumental rotation of L.O.T. to O.A.

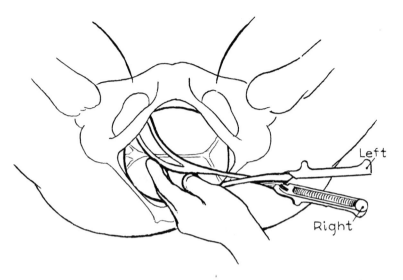

FIGURE 5–6. Wandering maneuver of anterior, or right, blade of Elliot forceps in application to L.O.T.

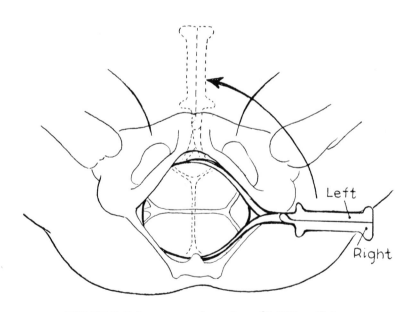

FIGURE 5–7. Instrumental rotation of L.O.T. to O.A.

The right blade is held in the right hand and introduced to the right side of the pelvis high up under the ramus, since the brow is more anterior than in L.O.A. owing to the transverse position (Fig. 5–5). The handle is then made to descend over an arc close to the left thigh while upward pressure at the heel of the blade is made with the middle finger of the left hand (Fig. 5–6). This maneuver throws the toe of the blade away from the anterior frontal eminence, wandering it around the head into place just in front of the anterior ear. As the handle of the wandering (right) blade approaches the handle of the posterior (left) blade, it will be found to be in a lower plane. In order to lock them, it will be necessary to elevate the handle of the right blade, causing the blade to slide farther up into the pelvis behind the symphysis until the handles meet. When locked, the handles lie in a plane obliquely to the left of the midline of the patient. This is necessary in order to bring the plane of the shanks one finger's breadth medial to the posterior fontanelle.

In the instrumental rotation, the steps are as follows: Flexion must be accomplished. The handles are moved in an arc, then depressed. With slight compression on the handles to fix the blades on the head, the handles are moved toward the midline, far enough to correct the flexion attitude. The handles are then rotated upward in a wide counterclockwise arc consistent with the pelvic curve of the instrument (Fig. 5–7). The object is to maintain a small arc with the toes of the blade, keeping the long axis of the head in the axis of the pelvis. As the 90-degree rotation is completed, the occiput comes to rest under the symphysis. The handles are depressed at completion to preserve or improve flexion. The application is again checked. If necessary, the blades are readjusted before traction in the axis of the pelvis. Traction is best performed with some form of axis traction instrument or attachment.

If the head will not rotate easily, it is probably because the handles are not being moved over a wide arc or the head is extended. These situations may be corrected. The head may be arrested with a minor relative disproportion at the level of least pelvic dimension, that is, the ischial spines. In that instance, the head may require slight upward displacement so that rotation may be accomplished closer to the plane of greatest pelvic dimension.

RIGHT OCCIPUT TRANSVERSE

In R.O.T. positions, the right, or posterior, blade is introduced first. This is done by holding the right blade in the right hand and applying it directly posterior to the right ear. The force exerted to introduce the blade is made mainly by the thumb pressing against the heel. The handle descends toward the right thigh so that the shank will be one finger's breadth medial to the posterior fontanelle. This avoids an application in the extended attitude. The handle may be held in this position by an assistant while the left blade is introduced high on the left side and wandered anteriorly in the usual manner. In right-sided positions, the handles must be crossed in order to lock them. In doing this, the finger guard may interfere with the crossing. One handle is pulled down while the other handle is pushed up, facilitating the crossing. A preliminary check of the application is made, and if it is found to be good, the head is flexed and rotated by carrying the handles clockwise over a wide arc to the anterior position. The application is rechecked. Readjustments are frequently found to be necessary in this position. They are made, and extraction is completed in the usual manner. If the application is not satisfactory after attempts at readjustment, the blades are removed and, after checking the position, they are reapplied.

SIX

Posterior Positions of the Occiput

Posterior positions are managed either by manual rotation or instrumental rotation to the anterior position, or by a combination of these two methods, when maternal or fetal indications exist for delivery. Special instruments (see following chapters) may be used. Less frequently, certain situations will be met in which delivery as an occiput posterior (O.P.) should be performed.

Manual Rotation—Left Occiput Posterior and Right Occiput Posterior

Manual rotation of a posterior head is accomplished in the same manner as the transverse head with the exception that the head must be rotated over a longer arc to the anterior position. The right hand is the rotating hand for a left occiput posterior (L.O.P.) (Fig. 6–1), and the left for a right occiput posterior (R.O.P.). After rotation to an anterior quadrant of the pelvis is accomplished manually, the thumb of the rotating hand is removed from the vagina while pressure is placed on the fundus by the assistant. The four fingers remain in place behind the posterior parietal bone in order to splint the head

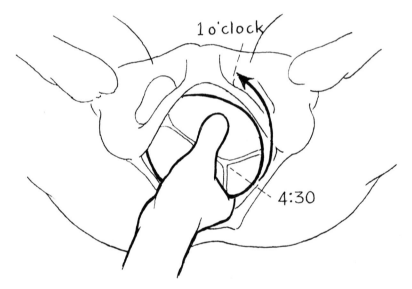

FIGURE 6–1. Manual rotation of L.O.P. to anterior with right hand.

and prevent it from rotating back to the transverse or posterior position while the posterior blade is being applied. The blade in left-sided positions of the occiput is the left blade. Its handle is held in the left hand, and it is inserted on the left side of the pelvis opposite the left ear. In right-sided positions, it is the right blade with the handle in the right hand. After the posterior blade has been placed in position opposite the posterior ear, the fingers of the rotating hand are removed from the vagina so that they can hold the handle of the anterior blade. This is introduced in the usual manner for an anterior position. Then the shanks are locked, the application is checked, and rotation to occiput anterior (O.A.) is completed. The application is rechecked, and any necessary readjustments are made before extraction is begun.

Combined Manual and Instrumental Rotation

If manual rotation of a posterior head cannot be accomplished beyond the transverse position, it may be completed instrumentally by applying the forceps as in a transverse arrest. The rotating hand is kept in place to act as a splint while the posterior blade is being applied (Fig. 6–2). The anterior blade is wandered around the brow by the elevating fingers at the heel as the handle is depressed well below the handle of the posterior blade. When the blade is in place behind the symphysis opposite the anterior ear, the handle is elevated to the locking position beneath the handle of the posterior blade. Completion of the rotation of the head instrumentally to the O.A. position is in a counterclockwise direction for left-sided positions. In right-sided positions, the direction is clockwise. After checking the application, traction is applied.

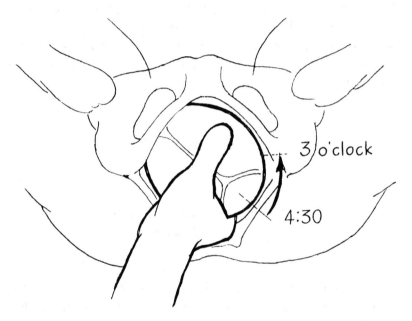

FIGURE 6–2. Manual rotation of L.O.P. to L.O.T. preparatory to application of Elliot type of forceps to L.O.T. using the wandering method for the anterior blade and completion of rotation to O.A. instrumentally.

Instrumental Rotation—Modified Scanzoni Maneuver— Left Occiput Posterior

The modified Scanzoni maneuver consists of complete instrumental rotation, with an Elliot type of forceps, of an occiput posterior to the anterior position. This is accomplished with a single maneuver, but a reapplication of the forceps is required for completion of the delivery.

An L.O.P. is considered as a right occiput anterior (R.O.A.), and the blades are applied accordingly. In the L.O.P. position, the right blade is held in the right hand and is applied first, over the left, or posterior, ear in the right side of the pelvis (Fig. 6–3). This is the first deviation from the cardinal point of the right blade to the right ear. After the right blade is applied, the left blade is taken in the left hand and applied to the left side of the pelvis to the right, or anterior, ear. The handles are crossed and the shanks locked (Fig. 6–4). A preliminary check should show the posterior fontanelle to be just *below* the plane of the shanks and the sagittal suture perpendicular to the plane of the shanks. The head is then rotated counterclockwise to the anterior position. The pelvic curve of the forceps makes it necessary to rotate the handles over a wide arc to keep the blades in the center of the pelvis, thereby avoiding obstruction or injury. Frequently, the head is extended, resulting in a deviation of the long axis of the head from the axis of the pelvis. If flexion is performed first, rotation will be made much easier because resistance will be decreased. If the widest part of the head is arrested at the plane of the ischial spines, it will be necessary to push it up 1 or 2 cm to bring it close to the plane of greatest pelvic dimension prior to rotation. Rotation at the inlet is not advised.

In L.O.P. positions, rotation is counterclockwise. After the handles are elevated in order to procure flexion, and after they are rotated in order to bring the occiput into the anterior oblique (left occiput anterior [L.O.A.]) diameter of the pelvis, the head is fixed in the new position by slight downward traction. Since the blades are now upside-down with the toes pointing posteriorly, they must be

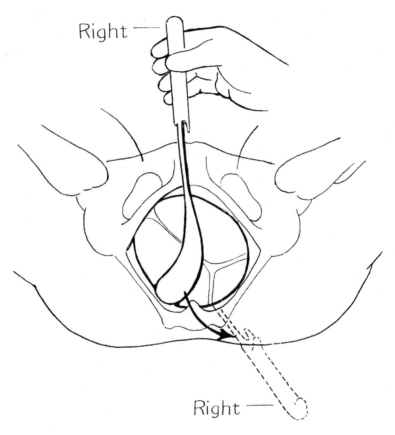

FIGURE 6–3. Insertion of posterior, or right, blade (Tucker-McLane), solid Elliot type in the first stage of the modified Scanzoni maneuver for instrumental rotation of L.O.P. to O.A.

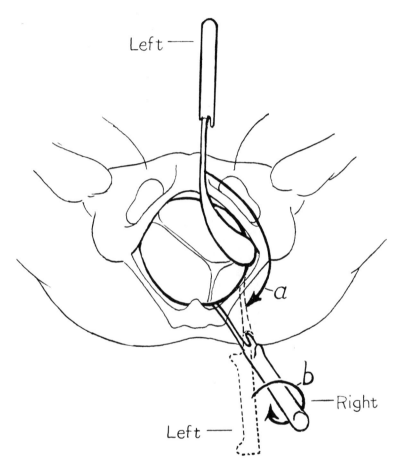

FIGURE 6–4. Insertion of anterior, or left, blade and crossing the handle, left over right, for locking in the first stage of the modified Scanzoni maneuver for L.O.P.

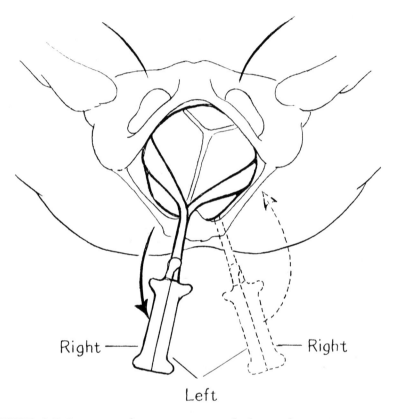

Right ——————   ———— Right

Left

FIGURE 6–5. Instrumental rotation, counterclockwise, from L.O.P. to anterior. This completes the first stage of the modified Scanzoni maneuver. The occiput is now anterior, but the blades are upside-down. The second stage involves removal, reinversion, and reapplication.

removed, inverted, and reapplied (Fig. 6–5). The posterior (right) blade, which is the one over the left ear, is temporarily retained in place to splint the head in the anterior position. The anterior blade is removed first, in a downward direction (Fig. 6–6). Since it is the left blade, it is reinserted between the head and the blade that is still in place opposite the left ear, as in the L.O.A. technique (Fig. 6–7). Following this, the right, or "splinting," blade is removed in a downward direction and reapplied over the right, or anterior, ear (Fig. 6–8). In the original Scanzoni maneuver, first introduced in the 19th century, after rotation of the head to the anterior quadrant of the pelvis, both blades are removed; the posterior blade is not left in place as a splint. They are then reapplied to the new anterior position. Frequently, the head rotates back toward the original position before reapplication can be made.

In performing this modified Scanzoni maneuver, it has been found that the Elliot type of forceps with overlapping shanks, especially the solid bladed Tucker-McLane, or the Luikart modification, is preferable. Less resistance is offered to application, rotation, and removal. Also, the Bill axis traction handle can be used as an aid to rotation as well as to traction. If desired, a different type of instrument with fenestrated blade may be used for the second application and for traction. It is very easy to slip a fenestrated blade between the head and a solid posterior splinting blade. A solid blade for rotation obviates the possibility of threading the reapplied blade through the fenestration of the splinting blade. Should this happen, it complicates the removal of the splinting blade. In this case, removal can be facilitated by withdrawing the blade along the surrounded shank, past the finger guard, to the end of the handle.

It is felt that the modified Scanzoni maneuver is preferable to the original maneuver in that the head is less likely to slip back to the transverse or posterior position due to the presence of the "splinting blade."

It must be emphasized that after rotation of the head to the anterior position in the first stage of this maneuver, the blades are upside-down, so that the pelvic curve is facing the sacrum. Therefore, removal of the blades must be accomplished by pulling downward on the handles toward the floor.

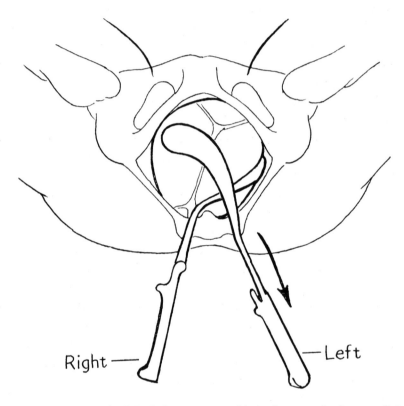

FIGURE 6–6. Removal of the left, or anterior, blade downward, after one fixing pull in this direction.

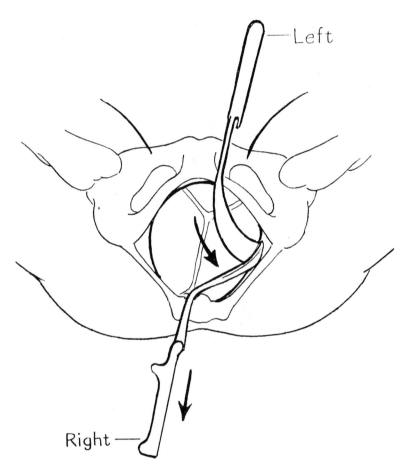

FIGURE 6–7. Reinversion and reinsertion of the left blade between the splinting right blade and the posterior, or left, ear as for L.O.A.

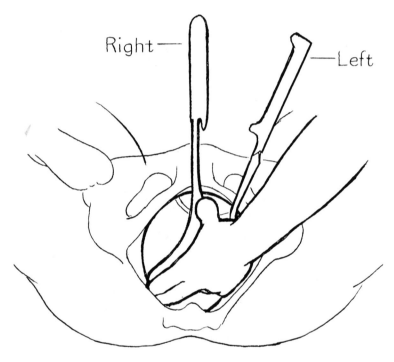

FIGURE 6–8. Reapplication of the right splinting blade to the anterior, or right, ear as in L.O.A., after removal in a downward direction and reinversion.

After the head has been rotated to the O.A. position, the reapplication is checked, and if found satisfactory, traction is begun (Fig. 6–9).

Scanzoni Maneuver—Right Occiput Posterior

The R.O.P. position is considered as an L.O.A., the blades are applied, and the head is rotated clockwise to the anterior quadrant. Removal and reapplication are similar to that of the L.O.P., except that in the second application, that is, to the new R.O.A. position, the handles must be crossed in order to lock them prior to traction.

Directly Posterior Heads (Occiput Posterior)

The occiput in the direct posterior position is treated similarly to the transverse or posterior oblique position except that it is rotated over a longer arc to the anterior position. The rotation may be manual or instrumental. Before attempting the rotation, it is necessary to know on which side the fetal back lies in order to know which way to rotate the head. This avoids the danger of injury to the neck from rotation in the wrong direction. The occiput should rotate through the side on which the back lies. Since a fetal position with the back posterior is rare, the back can be identified by abdominal palpation or ultrasound scan. With the back to the left, the rotation is counterclockwise using the same technique as in an L.O.P. With the back on the right side, rotation is clockwise as in an R.O.P. Following rotation, forceps application (or reapplication if a Scanzoni) and traction are performed as previously described.

The DeLee "Key in Lock" maneuver is a gradual instrumental rotation of an occiput posterior to the anterior by multiple readjustments of the forceps. This is accomplished with application as if the

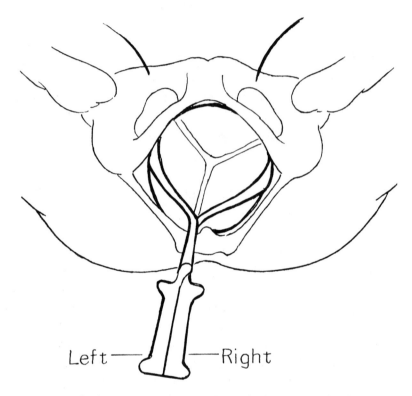

Left ———————————Right

FIGURE 6–9. The forceps are now properly applied and locked in the new L.O.A. position, ready for traction after completing rotation to O.A. The Bill handle should be added for traction.

posterior occiput were anterior. The instrument, classically a DeLee-Simpson, rotates the head through a 15- to 20-degree arc in the proper direction. It is then unlocked and readjusted and the movement repeated. The head is rotated in steps through 180 degrees with the instrument remaining in the anterior quadrants.

This maneuver has been popular in some areas but has generally been supplanted by methods that avoid asymmetrical stress to the fetal skull. It is presented as mainly of historical interest.

Delivery as an Occiput Posterior

Occasionally, in an anthropoid pelvis with a transverse diameter too narrow to permit anterior rotation, the posterior occiput should be delivered as such. The same procedure is used in a case of a marked funnel pelvis, usually android, with the occiput posterior molded into the outlet under a narrow arch.

For several reasons, delivery as a posterior is not a simple delivery. More force is required to accomplish descent of the occiput posterior. Since the head is being moved in an awkward direction, opposite to normal, the direction of the traction force is critical to avoid trauma to the head. With extension and molding of the head, the biparietal diameter may be at a higher level than anticipated. Considerably more soft tissue space is required, and a much greater risk exists for a fourth degree episiotomy extension. In our opinion, this should not be classified as an outlet forceps procedure, regardless of the station of the head.

An instrument employing the axis traction principle is preferred. The technique of application of forceps to an occiput posterior that is to be delivered without anterior rotation is similar to that for the first stage of the Scanzoni maneuver. Before locking the handles, they are depressed against the perineum until the shanks are close to the level of the posterior fontanelle. More effort in traction is necessary for delivery of an occiput posterior as such. After the anterior fontanelle appears under the symphysis, the head is delivered by flexion instead of by extension.

This discussion of posterior and transverse heads deals only with the utilization of the classical instruments. Many cases are handled much more efficiently with less manipulation and less effort if the operator uses a special instrument, such as the Kielland or Barton forceps or the more recent Laufe or Mann forceps. Certain modifications of classical instruments may also be used to manage posterior heads. For example, the Jacobs forceps (an Elliot type with solid blades attached to the shanks by a swivel joint), the LaBreck forceps

TABLE 6-1. **Operative Management of Occiput Posterior Positions**

1. MANUAL ROTATION TO O.A.
   A. Digital rotation

   } Followed by Simpson type; best with axis traction

   B. Manual rotation

2. COMBINED MANUAL AND INSTRUMENTAL ROTATION TO O.A.
   Wandering maneuver, Elliot-type forceps, after manual or digital rotation to transverse

3. INSTRUMENTAL ROTATION TO O.A.
   A. Classical instruments
      (a) Scanzoni maneuver (modified)
          Elliot-type forceps (solid blade: Tucker-McLane, Luikart)
      (b) DeLee "Key in Lock" maneuver *(not recommended)*
          Simpson-type forceps
   B. Modified classical instruments
      (a) Jacobs—Elliot type, solid blade
      (b) LaBreck—Simpson type, solid blade
      (c) Miseo—Elliot type, split universal joint
   C. Special instruments
      (a) Kielland
      (b) Barton
      (c) Laufe
      (d) Mann

4. DELIVER AS A POSTERIOR POSITION
   A. Android pelvis—selected cases (Simpson type, axis traction)
   B. Anthropoid pelvis—selected cases (Simpson type, axis traction)

Note: Internal podalic version, listed in the past as an alternative, is no longer considered to be acceptable.

(a Simpson type with solid blades and swivel jointed toes), and the Miseo forceps (an Elliot type with a split universal joint and parallel shanks) eliminate the necessity of removal and reapplication after rotation to anterior. (See chapters on special instruments.)

Operative Management of Occiput Posterior Positions

Table 6–1 details the operative management of occiput posterior positions.

SEVEN

*Special Instruments: Kielland Forceps**

In 1915, Christian Kielland of Norway presented his forceps to the obstetrical world. Although originally intended for application to heads in deep transverse arrest, this instrument is now used on posterior heads and occasionally on face and brow presentations. The instrument enjoys considerable popularity as a rotator in cases in which the occiput is not in one of the anterior quadrants of the pelvis. Some operators claim excellent results in elective low forceps use, and it has even been advocated as a substitute for Piper forceps to the aftercoming head.

In the past, the instrument was considered good for heads arrested in the higher levels of the pelvis, although this was not Kielland's original intention. Currently, this type of higher station procedure is not generally considered justifiable in view of the reported increased incidence of poor fetal results. In addition, the incidence of Kielland forceps failure is greater with higher stations of the head. Studies have indicated a greater neonatal morbidity and perinatal loss with Kielland rotation contrasted to vaginal delivery. However, vaginal delivery is not an available alternative when operative deliv-

*Note: Figures 7–1 through 7–4 and 7–12 through 7–17 depict application of the Kielland forceps with the biparietal diameter at the plane of the inlet. The transverse arrest as pictured would be a high forceps. The technique is no different at mid or low forceps levels.

ery is indicated. Comparing Kielland forceps results with those of cesarean section, a more relevant comparison, equal or superior results have been reported for the forceps operation. It should be noted that Kielland results do not differ significantly from nonrotational forceps or manual rotation followed by forceps delivery. In the author's opinion, however, the Kielland procedure has a less traumatic "feel" and is preferable.

Construction

This forceps has a slight pelvic curve that is backward, giving the instrument a bayonet-like shape. It has overlapping shanks with an extra long distance between the heels of the blades and the intersecting point of the shanks. The lock is a sliding one and is designed to correct for asynclitism. The inner surface of the blades is beveled to prevent injury to the fetal head. The knobs (or buttons) on each anterior surface of the finger guards are used to identify the anterior surface of the instrument and serve as a guide in the technique of application.

Advantages

A single accurate application without displacement of the head can be obtained by the inversion method because of the reverse pelvic curve.

The sliding lock principle permits adjustment of asynclitic heads and allows the locking of the handles at any level on the shank.

There is a semi axis traction pull due to the reverse pelvic curve.

The beveled inner surface of the blades minimizes facial injury.

The extra long distance between the heels of the blades and the intersecting point of the shanks lengthens the posterior portion of the cephalic curve of the instrument. This accommodates heads of different shapes and sizes regardless of molding.

The relatively straight design puts the shanks and handles close to the long axis of the fetal head. This also allows the toes of the blades to describe a very small circle during rotation along the long axis.

Disadvantages

In a flat pelvis with a high transverse arrest of a posterior parietal presentation, the Kielland forceps are distinctly contraindicated. When applied to this position, there is no available pelvic curve or axis traction. The mechanism of a flat pelvis requires descent of the head in the transverse diameter. A straight or forward-jutting upper sacrum presents the same problem, regardless of the station of the head in transverse arrest. The head must be drawn well past the point of deformity, in the transverse position, before it can be rotated to anterior.

In a male-type pelvis with a funnel outlet and a low symphysis, the reverse pelvic curve may cause injury to the posterior vaginal wall and perineum during extension. Also, during the same maneuver, elevation of the handles may bring that portion of the forceps connecting the blades with the shanks in contact with the pubic rami, possibly resulting in a periostitis. These potential problems are of particular significance if the operator thinks in terms of a classical instrument with its pronounced pelvic curve. Experimentation on the manikin quickly demonstrates the location of the toes and shanks during extension. Some operators prefer to remove the Kielland forceps after rotation and some descent have been accomplished. They substitute a suitable classical type of instrument with a good pelvic curve. They believe, probably without reason, that the Kielland forceps should be replaced with a better traction instrument for completion of the delivery.

Although this instrument has marked a great advance in obstetrical surgery, it is not a panacea. It can be dangerous if not properly used. The accidents that may happen with its misuse are perforation of the uterus, vesicovaginal fistula, perforation of the cul-de-sac, cer-

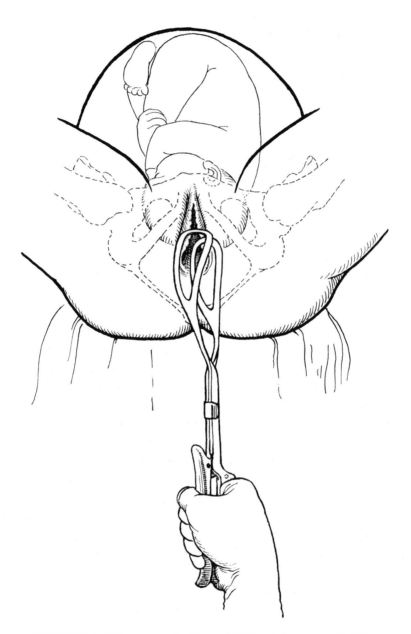

FIGURE 7–1. Orientation. Position of Kielland forceps on L.O.T.

vical and sulcus tear, and third- or fourth-degree laceration. However, all of these injuries may follow the use of any instrument, and some may be seen in spontaneous deliveries. The fault is not so much with the instrument as with the manner of its use.

Kielland Technique

LEFT OCCIPUT TRANSVERSE POSITION— DEEP TRANSVERSE ARREST

Application-Inversion Method ("Classical" Method)

Prior to the operative procedure, the urinary bladder should be emptied. Performance of the procedure on other than a delivery table is not advised; birthing room facilities are generally inadequate. The patient *must* be well down on the table, buttocks slightly overhanging the edge. If not, difficulty may be encountered in application and rotation. The table edge may prevent lowering of the handles to perpendicular to the plane of the pelvis at the level of the biparietal diameter.

Since the Kielland is a special type of instrument, the technique for the classical instrument of applying the posterior blade first is abandoned. Instead, the anterior blade is always applied first, preferably by Kielland's inversion method. In left-sided positions, the left ear is posterior and the right ear anterior. This requires the application of the right blade first. The blades are locked and held outside the pelvis, directed toward the patient in a position similar to that which they will assume when applied (Fig. 7–1). The knobs will be pointing in the direction of the occiput, toward the patient's left leg at 3 o'clock. The anterior blade is easily distinguished as the one on top, and it is found to be the right blade since there is no lock on its shank. This blade, after temporarily discarding the left blade, is held in an inverted manner, with the inner surface of the cephalic curve facing upward and the shank 45 degrees above the horizontal.

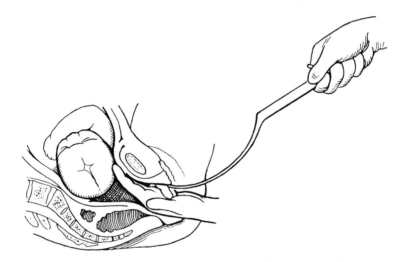

FIGURE 7–2. Introduction of anterior, or right, blade of Kielland forceps to anterior, or right, ear in L.O.T. by the inversion method.

The blade, the handle of which is held in the right hand, rests in the palm of the left hand, the tips of the middle and index fingers of which are inserted under the symphysis, anterior to the head (Fig. 7–2). The toe is passed directly under the symphysis and is guided by the fingertips. The cervix, when fully dilated and retracted, should not be palpable. Should obstruction be met when the toe has passed the fingertips, gentle advancing pressure with a slight pump handle motion may be employed, feeling for the plane of least resistance. The object is to maintain the toe close to the head until the fenestration has disappeared from sight. Excessive force during this maneuver is ill advised. By this time, the handle has been lowered in the midline to the level of the horizontal. When the heel of the blade has passed under the symphysis, the handle has been further depressed to an angle of about 45 degrees below the horizontal, and the fenestration has reached its destination opposite the anterior cheek. The toe of the instrument may now be seen elevating the lower abdominal wall through the lower uterine segment. The "elbow" of the blade at the leading end of the shank should be close to the introitus, bringing a narrower diameter of the instrument between the head and symphysis. The higher the head is in the pelvis, the lower the handle will be below the horizontal, and the further into the uterus the blade will have to be inserted (Fig. 7–3).

Since the blade has been introduced in the inverted manner, its cephalic curve is directed away from the head toward the anterior wall of the uterus. It must now be rotated so that its cephalic curve will coincide with the curve of the head. Rotation of the blade is on its own axis *away* from the occiput toward the midline and toward the knob. This is accomplished by the right hand grasping the handle and thumb pressing against the side of the finger guard opposite the knob, turning it counterclockwise with a twist of the wrist over an arc of 180 degrees, until the knob points toward 3 o'clock. As the rotation is being completed, the handle is depressed slightly in order to follow the plane of least resistance (Fig. 7–4). If the blade is rotated in the wrong direction, that is, *toward* the occiput, the high point of the toe rubs against the anterior wall of the uterus and might cause damage.

Greater force is not used if resistance to rotation is encountered. The blade may not be inside the cervix, or if it is inside the cervix, it

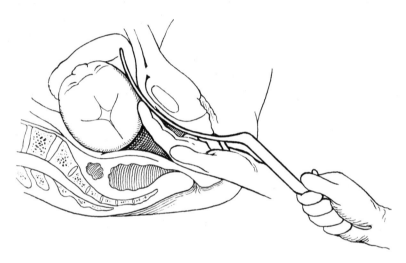

FIGURE 7–3. Anterior, or right, blade of Kielland forceps in place opposite the anterior, or right, ear in L.O.T. with its cephalic curve directed away from the head.

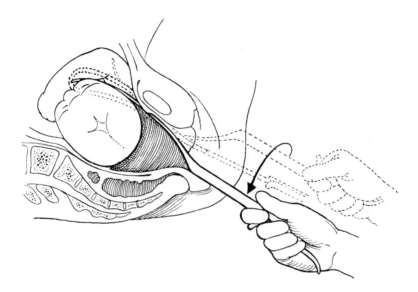

FIGURE 7–4. Rotation of anterior, or right, blade of Kielland forceps counter-clockwise in L.O.T. so its cephalic curve will coincide with the curve of the head.

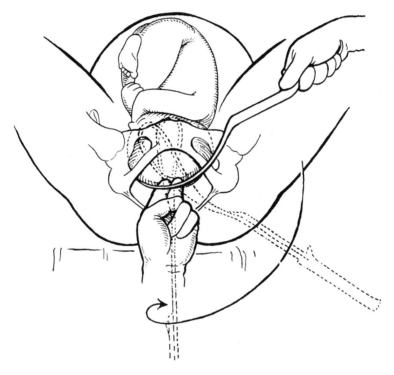

FIGURE 7–5. The "wandering maneuver" for application of the anterior, or right, blade of the Kielland forceps to the anterior, or right, ear of L.O.T.

may be either not far enough, or too far inside the uterus. Resistance to both introduction and rotation may also be encountered if a low contraction ring is present. Introduction of the blade carries more risk than rotation because in rotation the beveled edge will not cut the uterus, but will lift it away from the head. In introduction, the toe could be forced through a thin lower uterine segment.

Wandering Method of Application

If it is impossible to rotate the anterior blade after it is inside the uterus, the inversion method of application of the Kielland forceps is abandoned. The anterior blade is then applied by the gliding, or wandering, maneuver, carrying it around the face to the anterior ear, as in the classical instrument (Fig. 7–5). If the head is well flexed, interference often is encountered in wandering the blade around the side of the face. This may be avoided by reversing the maneuver and wandering the same blade, *upside-down,* around the side of the occiput (Fig. 7–6). In the belief that the wandering method is less hazardous than Kielland's inversion method, some operators prefer to use it exclusively. However, if the inversion method is not used, the same disadvantages accompanying the use of the wandering method with the classical instrument are encountered.

Direct Method of Application

Infrequently, the head is so low in the pelvis in the transverse position that it is difficult—or even impossible—to apply the anterior blade of the Kielland forceps by either the inversion or the wandering method. This situation is encountered when the head is near the outlet in the transverse position with an anterior parietal presentation. Because of the asynclitism and depth of engagement, the anterior ear can be palpated vaginally just behind the symphysis. Here a direct application is preferred.

In the direct application, the anterior blade—the right blade for a left occiput transverse (L.O.T.) and the left blade for a right occiput transverse (R.O.T.)—is applied directly under the symphysis to the

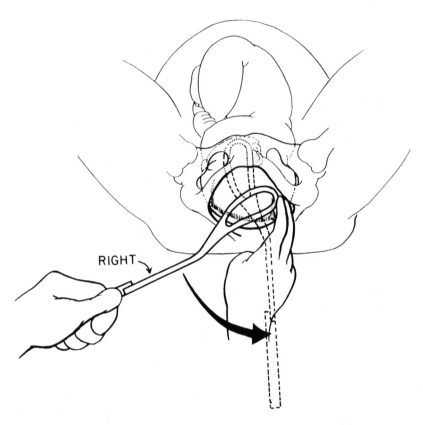

FIGURE 7–6. The "reverse wandering maneuver" for application of the anterior, or right, blade of the Kielland forceps held, upside-down, in the left hand, inserted to the left side of the pelvis and wandered, counterclockwise, to the anterior, or right, ear of L.O.T. with flexed head.

anterior ear (Fig. 7–7). The approach is from below upward, with the handle pointing toward the floor below the edge of the table. The concave, beveled surface of the blade is in contact with the anterior parietal bone, and the toe is directed under the symphysis toward the anterior ear. With gentle upward insertion, the blade slides up to the desired location on the anterior cheek.

Posterior Blade

Following application of the anterior blade by the appropriate application technique, the posterior, or left, blade is introduced. It is always introduced posteriorly between the shank of the anterior blade and the patient's right thigh, regardless of the method of application of the anterior blade. This obviates the necessity of crossing the handles in order to lock them. Guiding fingers, palm up, are introduced inside the vagina posterior to the head. The blade, with the cephalic curve up, is passed directly behind the head along the palmar surface of the guiding hand (Fig. 7–8). More difficulty may be encountered with the introduction of this blade than the anterior, owing to the obstruction that may be caused by the promontory. If resistance is met, the handle of the posterior blade may be moved up and down, with a jiggling motion as it is inserted, in order to bring the toe inside the retracted cervix and keep it hugging the head. Should resistance be met in the midline, the direction of the toe can be shifted slightly to either side of the midline to avoid an obstruction. When the blade is opposite the posterior, or left, ear, the shanks are locked (Fig. 7–9). The sliding lock permits this at any level on the shank. One handle may be at a higher level than the other owing to an asynclitic application. Traction is made on the finger guard that is nearer the perineum. Simultaneously, pressure is applied in the opposite direction to the other finger guard until the handles are equalized, thus correcting the asynclitism. If the posterior blade cannot be inserted far enough to permit locking, the use of extra force should be avoided. Downward traction on the handle of the anterior blade against the head should cause the latter to descend on the inclined plane of the cephalic curve of the posterior blade far enough to allow the handles to be locked. After a preliminary check of the application, the head is rotated counterclockwise 90 degrees to the occiput anterior position.

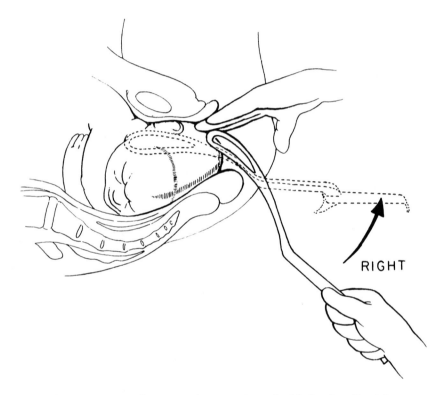

RIGHT

FIGURE 7–7. "Direct application" of anterior, or right, blade of Kielland forceps to anterior, or right, ear of L.O.T. Vertex near perineum with marked anterior parietal presentation.

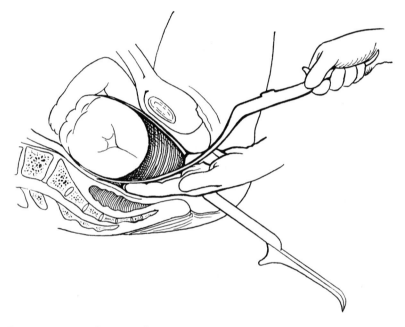

FIGURE 7–8. Introduction of posterior, or left, blade of Kielland forceps directly to the posterior, or left, ear in L.O.T.

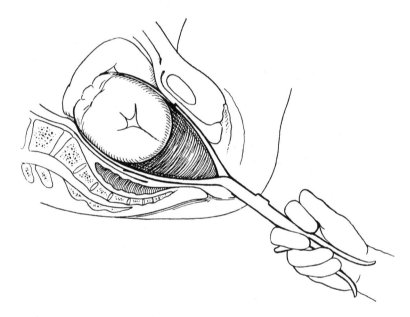

FIGURE 7–9. Kielland forceps applied to L.O.T.

Rotation

Because of the reverse pelvic curve of the Kielland forceps, rotation is not over a wide arc, but is almost directly on the axis of the shanks, with depression of the handles at the completion of the turn (Fig. 7–10).

The rotational force required should not be great. The novice is usually amazed that the thumb and index finger on the finger guards can easily accomplish most rotations. A check that the head is rotating with the forceps can be made with a finger resting on the scalp if visual control is not feasible during the procedure.

If resistance to rotation of the head is encountered in a normal pelvis, it is most commonly due to a failure to depress the handles to the proper level, namely, perpendicular to the plane of the pelvis at the level of the biparietal diameter. Lower the handles for a higher biparietal.

Extension of the head obstructs rotation along its long axis. Flexion is accomplished by readjustment of the forceps so that the plane of the shanks is within a finger's breadth anterior to the posterior fontanelle. Then the handles are lightly compressed and carried to the midline. Rotation can then be attempted.

On occasion, rotation at the level of application may be difficult. In order to bring the biparietal diameter to a different level in the pelvis, downward traction for 1 to 2 cm should be tried, rather than losing station. Should easy rotation be unsuccessful, the head should be displaced upward to a centimeter above its original station. This should bring the biparietal diameter well into the plane of greatest pelvic dimension, and rotation should proceed.

Note: In earlier editions, the warning was given that "traction with the head in the transverse diameter of the inlet is contraindicated if the bulge of the anterior blade is above the symphysis, because it exerts force against the symphysis and the bladder. There is no present day reason to use high forceps, so this statement becomes unnecessary. Similarly, displacement of the head to the inlet or higher, in order to accomplish rotation, is a dangerous procedure. Subsequent traction is on an unengaged head. The risk of such a procedure makes cesarean section the preferable route.

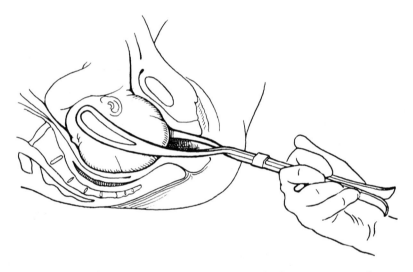

FIGURE 7–10. Kielland application after counterclockwise rotation of L.O.T. to
O.A.

If a situation is met in which rotation cannot be accomplished, the operator must eschew obstinacy and particularly the use of greater force. The forceps may be removed and the overall situation re-evaluated. Reapplication may then be tried. Alternatively, the delivery may be accomplished with the Barton forceps, particularly if shortened anteroposterior diameters exist. In that case, traction in the transverse can bring the head past the point of obstruction before anterior rotation. Otherwise, delivery should be abdominal. Unsuccessful attempts with Kielland forceps are not associated with increased fetal morbidity, provided excessive force is avoided.

Traction

After rotation has been completed, the application is rechecked, and if found to be correct, traction is begun. Traction, which is a backward pull in the direction of the handles, may be aided by the Saxtorph or Pajot maneuver. The finger guards are encircled by the middle and index fingers of the dominant hand, with the palm up (Fig. 7–11).

The slight reverse pelvic curve of the forceps gives a semi axis traction pull. Thus, the direction of traction is considerably lower than with the classical forceps. If the biparietal diameter is in the plane of greatest pelvic dimension, the direction of traction should be about 45 degrees below the horizontal. Voluntary bearing down by the patient is always used to assist in traction, assuming this is feasible. An episiotomy may be performed at an appropriate time. Lowering of the legs may give further relief of tension on the perineum.

As the posterior fontanelle is delivered, the handles are gradually elevated to the horizontal during traction. The technique is similar to that of the classical instrument, except that it is important never to elevate the handles of the Kielland forceps above the horizontal. The backward pelvic curve of the blade may cause a sulcus tear. In order to gain more extension, a special maneuver may be employed. Pressure is applied to the fundus by the assistant to keep the head from receding. The handles are unlocked and depressed, one at a time, toward the floor, so that the plane of the shanks is two or three

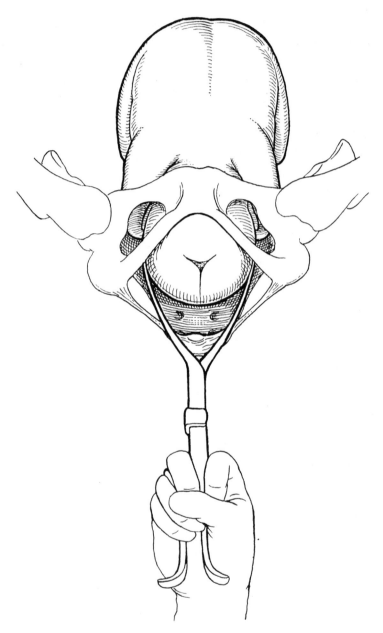

FIGURE 7–11. Traction on O.A. after anterior rotation with the Kielland forceps.

fingers below the posterior fontanelle. The handles are then locked and elevated to the horizontal while slight traction is being made. This maneuver causes extension of the head without digging the toes of the blades into the sulci. It may be repeated in order to gain the required extension for the performance of the Ritgen maneuver. The blades are then removed, taking the top, or right, blade off first, following the technique of the classical type of instrument. If difficulty is experienced in removing the blades, rather than use undue force, it is advisable to deliver the head with one or both blades still in place.

RIGHT OCCIPUT TRANSVERSE POSITION

In the R.O.T. position, the left ear is anterior, so the left blade, which is the anterior blade and has the lock on it, is applied first (Fig. 7–12). It is applied under the symphysis, and into the uterus, as already described (Figs. 7–13, 7–14). It is rotated in a clockwise direction away from the occiput toward the midline, until the knob on the handle points toward the patient's right leg at 9 o'clock (Fig. 7–15). The posterior blade is applied between the shank of the anterior blade and the right thigh, as in the L.O.T. position (Figs. 7–16, 7–17). The head is rotated clockwise to the anterior position. The application is rechecked, and if found satisfactory, traction is applied and delivery is completed (Fig. 7–18).

KIELLAND FORCEPS APPLIED
TO POSTERIOR POSITIONS

Left Occiput Posterior Position

Assuming that the posterior fontanelle is at 4 o'clock, the blades are held in front of the patient, locked in the position that they will occupy when applied. Therefore, the knobs point toward 4 o'clock. The anterior (right) blade is grasped, and the posterior (left) blade is temporarily discarded. The anterior blade is introduced under the symphysis to the anterior, or right, ear in the same manner as when applied to a direct transverse position. After insertion, it is rotated away from the occiput and toward the midline in a counterclockwise

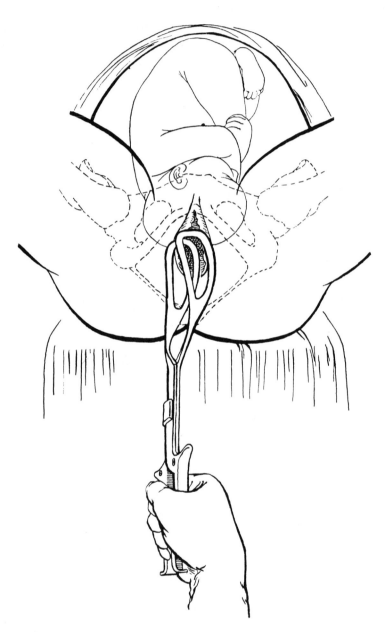

FIGURE 7–12. Orientation for position of Kielland forceps on R.O.T.

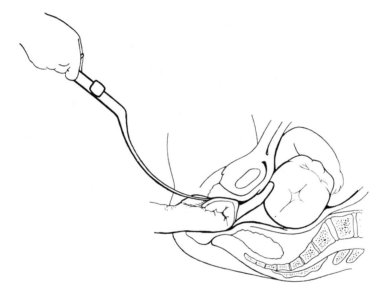

FIGURE 7–13. Insertion of anterior, or left, blade of Kielland forceps to anterior, or left, ear of R.O.T. by the inversion method.

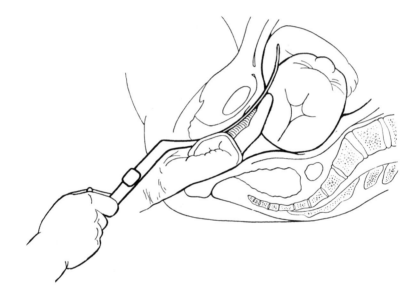

FIGURE 7–14. Anterior, or left, blade of Kielland forceps opposite anterior, or left, ear of R.O.T.

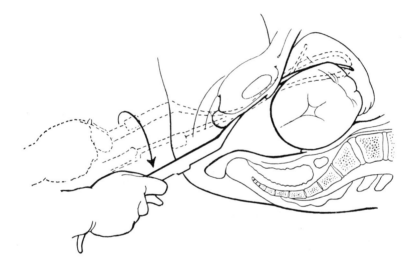

FIGURE 7–15. Clockwise rotation in R.O.T. of anterior, or left, blade of Kielland forceps so that its cephalic curve will coincide with the curve of the head.

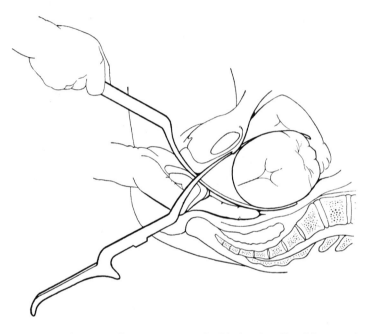

FIGURE 7–16. Application of posterior, or right, blade of Kielland forceps directly to posterior, or right, ear of R.O.T.

direction, until the knob on the finger guard points toward 4 o'clock. The rotation in this instance is over an arc of about 135 degrees to the posterior oblique position of the head, instead of the 180-degree arc to the transverse position.

Resistance to rotation of the inverted anterior blade, which is inside the cervix, may often be overcome by carrying the handle away from the midline toward the occiput. The posterior blade is then inserted, introduced posteriorly in the oblique diameter, parallel to the sagittal suture, so that it will pass directly to the posterior ear. Then, after locking the handles, asynclitism is corrected by pulling down on the finger guard that is nearer the patient's perineum and by pushing up on the other. The head is then flexed and rotated counterclockwise over an arc of about 135 degrees to the anterior position. The application is checked, and traction is applied as previously described.

Right Occiput Posterior Position

The occiput is assumed to be at 8 o'clock. The right ear is posterior and the left ear is anterior, so the left, or anterior, blade, the one with the lock, is introduced first. The introduction is the same as in the R.O.T. position; however, after clockwise rotation away from the occiput, the knob on the handle points to 8 o'clock instead of pointing to 9 o'clock, as in the transverse position. The posterior, or right, blade is inserted posteriorly as in the left occiput posterior (L.O.P.) position, except that it follows the opposite oblique diameter parallel to the sagittal suture. The handles are locked, asynclitism is corrected, and the head is flexed and rotated clockwise to the anterior position. Extraction is performed in the usual manner.

Direct Occiput Posterior Positions

The obstetrician is frequently confronted with the situation in which the occiput engages in a posterior position or rotates posteriorly during the course of labor. If the decision is made to deliver with a forceps rotation, the Kielland forceps procedure is considered supe-

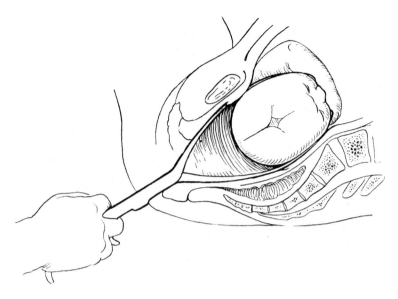

FIGURE 7–17. Kielland forceps applied to R.O.T.

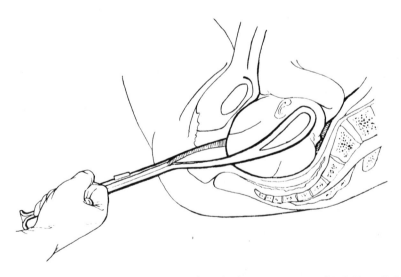

FIGURE 7–18. Kielland application after clockwise rotation of R.O.T. to O.A.

rior to the Scanzoni. A single accurate application with an instrument designed for rotation and traction is felt to be less traumatic.

With a direct occiput posterior, one must be certain of the location of the fetal back in order to avoid rotation in the wrong direction. Although observation of position during labor and abdominal palpation are helpful, a quick ultrasound scan should resolve any question.

With the occiput posteriorly and the sagittal suture pointed between 5 and 7 o'clock, the inversion method of application is not used. Instead, a reverse, or upside-down, direct application is employed with the knobs facing the floor. The approach is from below, upward, with the handles at an angle of about 45 degrees below the horizontal. The operator, sitting or kneeling, applies the blades directly to the sides of the head. In order to facilitate locking, the right blade, the one with the lock, is always introduced first. It goes to the left side of the pelvis, opposite the right ear.

If the occiput is directly posterior, the forceps are held with the toes inverted, the knobs pointing downward, locked in the position of application. The right blade is taken in the left hand and introduced from below the right thigh of the patient, upward at a 45-degree angle. The toe passes directly to the right side of the fetal head, on the left side of the mother's pelvis (Fig. 7–19). The left blade is then taken in the right hand and inserted from below the patient's left thigh to the left side of the head. The blades are locked, and the application is checked. If necessary, the head is flexed by elevating the handles. Rotation is accomplished by turning the handles through 180 degrees in the direction of the fetal back. The technique is the same as in rotation from occiput transverse. The usual direction of the handles is in the midline at about 45 degrees below the horizontal, but it is higher with a lower head.

When the occiput is found to be a few degrees away from direct occiput posterior (O.P.), that is, toward 5 or 7 o'clock, the application is similar. The direct application is adjusted in the proper direction to maintain the blades perpendicular to the sagittal suture.

The upside-down direct application technique should not be used unless the station of the head is well down in the pelvis. If the head is at mid station or higher, the reverse pelvic curve on the Kielland forceps interferes with application. Also, as previously

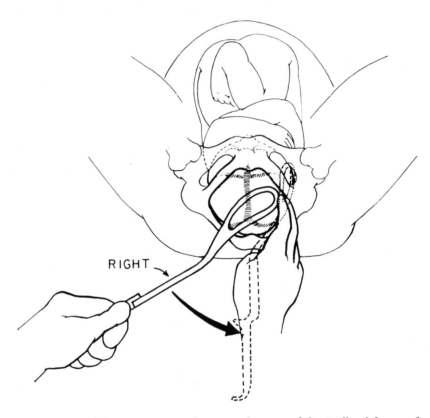

RIGHT

FIGURE 7–19. The "upside-down direct" application of the Kielland forceps for O.P. The right blade, with the anterior surface of its shank pointing downward, is held in the left hand and introduced to the left side of the patient's pelvis directly to the right ear.

noted, a fetal head at higher station would argue against a forceps procedure. Some would consider a vacuum extractor, although abdominal delivery would probably be the procedure of choice.

Kielland Forceps Applied to Face Presentation

The use of forceps in the uncommon face presentation is somewhat limited. Most authors follow the dictum, "If a face is making progress and there is no fetal heart rate abnormality, leave it alone." With greater extension of the fetal head, the biparietal diameter is higher in relation to the leading bony point. The ultimate in extension is past a brow, to a face presentation. In consequence, the biparietal diameter, and thus the effective level of forceps application, is higher than the operator anticipates. Lowest level forceps to a mentum anterior has been associated with excellent results. In other situations, namely, a higher head and transverse or posterior mentum positions, results appear less favorable. That technique is presented for the case in which a trial at vaginal delivery appears indicated. The same Kielland forceps precautions, contraindications, and maneuvers apply as in previous occiput techniques.

ANTERIOR CHIN

In face presentation with the chin anterior, a direct application to the sides of the face is made with the Kielland or a classical instrument, preferably with axis traction. Since the chin replaces the occiput as the presenting part, another exception to one of the cardinal points of forceps application arises. The left blade, instead of being applied to the left side of the face, is applied to the right side. The left blade, held in the left hand, is inserted into the left side of the vagina over the right ear. The right blade, held in the right hand, is inserted into the right side of the vagina over the left ear. The application is checked, using the mouth as the reference point in place of the posterior fontanelle. Traction is made downward, preserving complete

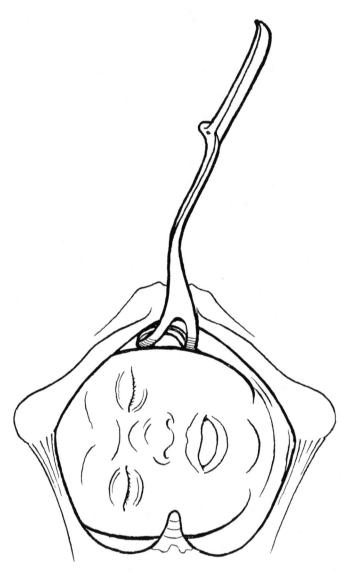

FIGURE 7–20. Insertion of anterior, or right, blade of Kielland forceps to anterior, or left, ear of a face presentation, L.M.T., by the inversion method.

extension until the chin passes under the symphysis. The handles are then elevated gradually to the horizontal with traction, so that the occiput is delivered over the perineum and the head is delivered by flexion.

TRANSVERSE CHIN

Rotation of a mentum transverse cannot and should not be performed unless the head is well down in the pelvis.

In all face presentations, the chin takes the place of the occiput, and the Kielland forceps is applied accordingly. In a *right mentum transverse (R.M.T.) position*, the application is the same as for an R.O.T. The left, or anterior, blade is inserted first, under the symphysis to the right, or anterior, ear, by the inversion method. Rotation of the left blade is clockwise toward the midline away from the chin. The right blade is then inserted directly posteriorly, to the left, or posterior, ear. The shanks are locked, and clockwise rotation of the chin toward 12 o'clock is performed, bringing it under the symphysis. Downward traction is made after checking the application. The head is delivered by flexion, following the chin under the symphysis.

In a *left mentum transverse (L.M.T.) position*, the application is the same as for an L.O.T. Therefore, the right blade is inserted under the symphysis above the left, or anterior, ear (the second exception to the cardinal rule of left blade to left ear). The toe of the blade is carried into the uterus in the inverted manner (Fig. 7–20). The blade is then rotated counterclockwise away from the chin, toward the midline and toward the knob (Fig. 7–21). The left blade is inserted directly posteriorly, and the shanks are locked. Rotation of the head in a counterclockwise direction brings the chin under the symphysis. Depression of the handles at the completion of rotation assures complete extension. Traction and delivery are accomplished as in an anterior chin position (Fig. 7–22).

If the inversion method of application is thought inadvisable, the anterior blade may be applied by the wandering maneuver.

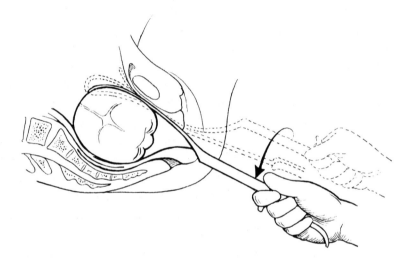

FIGURE 7–21. Counterclockwise rotation of an anterior, or right, blade of the Kielland forceps to anterior, or left, ear of a face presentation, L.M.T., so that its cephalic curve will coincide with the curve of the head.

POSTERIOR CHIN

A posterior chin cannot be delivered as such with any degree of safety. If the chin is in a direct or oblique posterior position, vaginal delivery is usually not advised. The Kielland technique would be similar to that for an occiput posterior, substituting the mentum as the point of reference. The head is usually at a higher level, however, and cesarean section is a preferable alternative.

Brow Presentation

The Kielland forceps has been used occasionally for brow presentations. When used, the head is either flexed or extended in order to change the brow to an occiput or face presentation. The pivot point of the fetal head in brow presentations is not in the center of the forceps blades. Therefore, traction tends to increase the extension. Also, the fetal head extension gives a higher biparietal diameter in relation to the leading bony point. Poor results attending forceps delivery of brow presentations are common. Cesarean section is usually preferable.

Methods of Application of Kielland Forceps

The methods of application of Kielland forceps are listed in the order of frequency of indicated use, as follows:

1. *Inversion: For transverse and posterior positions except the direct O.P.* This is indicated in most anthropoid and android pelves, plus all gynecoid pelves. The contraindications are a platypelloid pelvis, especially one with a posterior parietal presentation; a straight or deformed sacrum shortening the anteroposterior diameter of mid pelvis; unavoidable resistance or obstruction to the use of this ma-

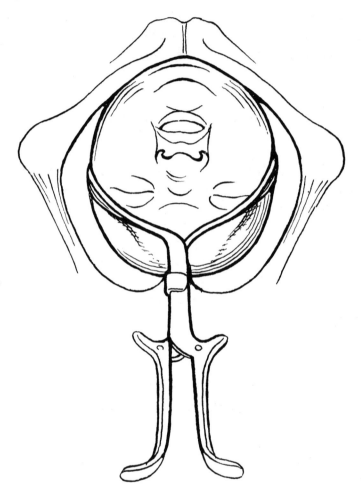

FIGURE 7–22. Application of Kielland forceps to an anterior chin, ready for traction, after counterclockwise rotation of a face presentation, L.M.T. to M.A.

neuver; a direct occiput posterior position; a transverse position with an anterior parietal presentation well down in the pelvis.

2. *Wandering: For transverse positions.* This is indicated when the inversion method meets resistance. Since the head is usually incompletely flexed, the anterior blade is wandered around the side of the face. The contraindications are the same as those given for the inversion method.

2A. *Reverse Wandering:* When the head is well flexed, the anterior blade is wandered around the side of the occiput, thereby avoiding resistance caused by the forehead.

3. *Direct: For transverse positions in the outlet with an anterior parietal presentation.* The anterior blade is inserted directly (not inverted) to the anterior cheek and ear, which can often be palpated behind the symphysis. The direct method is rarely used on anterior positions because a classical type of forceps is preferable.

3A. *Upside-Down Direct: For direct occiput posterior positions near the outlet.* The blades are applied upside-down, directly to the sides of the head. This method is used with caution on android and anthropoid pelves. Some have insufficient room for anterior rotation of the occiput. These may require delivery as an occiput posterior.

The standard method of application in most instances is the "inversion method." This provides the main advantage of the Kielland, namely, a single, accurate application without displacement. It can be accomplished without undue hazard because of the construction of the instrument.

The term "classical method," instead of the more specific term "inversion method," has crept into the literature and into case histories. This term is not favored because it has led to confusion, being misinterpreted as referring to the classical method used for applying a classical type of forceps. When referring to the Kielland, it suggests the "wandering method" and not the standard procedure by inversion.

EIGHT

Special Instruments: Barton Forceps*

Dr. Lyman G. Barton of Plattsburg, N.Y., designed his forceps for application to heads arrested in the transverse diameter of the inlet, especially those with a posterior parietal presentation. The instrument may be used to advantage in deep transverse arrest, oblique posterior position, and, rarely, in face presentation. The forceps was presented in 1925. Although in most areas of modern obstetrics the usage of the instrument is infrequent, there is a place for it. We find that those cases are usually ones in which there are relative contraindications to the use of the Kielland forceps. Those contraindications are most often the indication for the Barton forceps, namely, short anteroposterior diameters in the pelvis.

Construction

One blade is attached to the shank by a hinge, making it flexible over an arc of 90 degrees. The other blade has a deep cephalic curve. The

---

*Note: Figures 8–1 through 8–8 depict application of the Barton forceps with the biparietal diameter at the plane of the inlet. The transverse arrest as pictured would be a high forceps. The technique is no different at mid or low forceps levels.

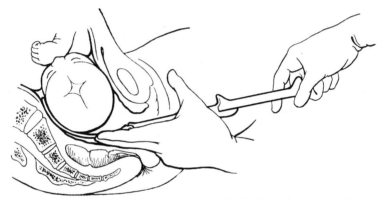

FIGURE 8–1. Introduction of the first, or hinged, blade of the Barton forceps for L.O.T. with *partial extension* (both fontanelles can be felt with equal ease). The handle is held in the *right* hand and the index and middle fingers of the left hand are at the heel, after guiding the toe of the blade directly posterior to the head.

blades are solid and are attached to the shanks laterally at an angle of about 50 degrees, so that when the forceps is held in the anterior position, there is no pelvic curve. However, when it is rotated over an arc of 90 degrees to the transverse position, the angle of attachment of the blades to the shanks forms a perfect pelvic curve. The lock is of the sliding type. There is a separate traction handle that can be applied to give axis traction. The use of the traction handle is advised since it greatly facilitates the mechanics of use of the instrument. It also aids the operator to think in terms of the long axis of the head. This is important considering the Barton forceps' difference from classical instruments.

Advantages

The thin hinged blade affords an easy and accurate application by the wandering maneuver to transverse heads, particularly those having a posterior parietal presentation. The hinge allows the blade to be wandered around the head into place in front of the anterior ear, behind the symphysis. With a fixed blade, it is impossible to obtain this application to a posterior parietal presentation because the anterior parietal bone overrides the symphysis, particularly at higher station.

The sliding lock allows for correction of asynclitism, as locking can be accomplished at any level on the shank.

The lateral attachment of the blades to the shanks forms a perfect pelvic curve when applied to a transverse head. Thus, descent may be accomplished safely by traction in this diameter before rotation.

The traction handle gives good axis traction.

The most important indication for the use of this instrument is a flat pelvis with a head arrested at mid pelvis in the transverse diameter. Here, the only instrument that can be used with safety is one that has a flexible blade attachment that allows the blades to conform to the curve of the pelvis when applied to a transverse head. This permits traction in the transverse diameter. This applies also to pelves with a straight or forward-jutting upper sacrum, thus shortening the anteroposterior diameter of the mid pelvis.

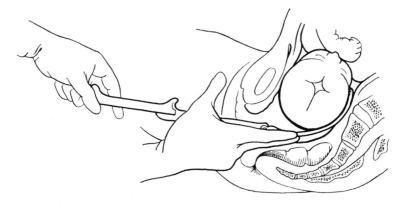

FIGURE 8–2. Introduction of the first, or hinged, blade of the Barton forceps for R.O.T. with *partial extension*. The handle is held in the *left* hand and the index and middle fingers of the right hand are at the heel, after guiding the toe of the blade directly posterior to the head.

Disadvantages

A disadvantage attached to this instrument is the possibility of its slipping when used on a difficult case, owing to its lightness, flexibility, and smooth blades. Another disadvantage is that it may be necessary to remove the forceps after rotation and apply a classical-type instrument for the extraction. The reason for this is that after rotation to anterior, the Barton has no pelvic curve, without which extension over the perineum requires much more effort for delivery. Also after rotation, the handles are directed obliquely away from the long axis of the patient. This makes traction awkward, even with the axis traction handle.

The Barton forceps is undesirable in android and anthropoid pelves. Here, because of a transverse contraction, descent of the head should occur in or near the anteroposterior diameter. The Barton is constructed to give traction for descent in the transverse position. Immediate rotation followed by traction with this instrument, in these pelves, requires much more effort. As a result, injuries to the vagina and avoidable stress to the fetal skull may be anticipated.

When planning instrumental delivery of a head arrested in a pelvis with short anteroposterior diameters, one should also consider the recently reported increased incidence of shoulder dystocia in such cases, particularly following a prolonged second stage of labor. An estimate of fetal size should be included in the decision to proceed vaginally. Naturally, the operator should be familiar with the treatment of shoulder dystocia.

Technique

TRANSVERSE POSITIONS—
LEFT OCCIPUT TRANSVERSE AND
RIGHT OCCIPUT TRANSVERSE

The hinged blade is the anterior blade and is always introduced first. Introduction is posteriorly, or in a posterior quadrant, prior to the wandering maneuver to bring it anterior (Figs. 8–1, 8–2). Fetal atti-

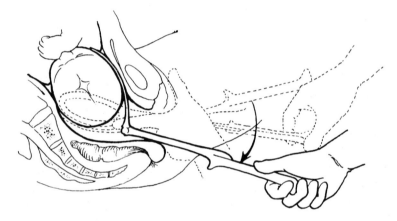

FIGURE 8–3. The hinged Barton blade has been "wandered" by the index and middle fingers of the *left* hand, around the right side of the pelvis over the *face* of an *extended* L.O.T., to the anterior, or right, ear behind the symphysis. The *right* hand on the hinged handle changes its level as the blade approaches the anterior ear.

tude is important to wandering. If the head is extended, less resistance is usually encountered if the blade is wandered over the face (Fig. 8–3). With a well-flexed head, there should be less resistance to wandering over the occiput (Fig. 8–4). In any case, should an obstruction be met, the opposite side can be tried.

With the anterior blade in place and held by an assistant, the posterior blade is then inserted directly posteriorly between the handle of the anterior blade and the patient's right thigh. The deep scoop of the posterior blade keeps the toe of the blade hugging the head, thereby avoiding the posterior lip of the cervix and the promontory of the sacrum (Figs. 8–5, 8–6). The anterior blade usually is farther up in the pelvis than the posterior. However, no difficulty in locking is encountered since the sliding lock permits this maneuver to be carried out at any level on the shank. In locking, the handle of the posterior blade, which is at or above the level of the horizontal, should not be depressed. Instead, the handle of the anterior hinged blade should be elevated to meet it. Traction on the under finger guard, combined with the modified Pajot maneuver, simultaneously corrects asynclitism and lowers the station of the head (Figs. 8–7, 8–8, 8–9, 8–10). The application should be checked prior to significant traction, however. The sagittal suture should be perpendicular to the plane of the shanks. The hinge level should be one finger's breadth medial to the posterior fontanelle. The traction handle is next attached to the shanks between the finger guard and the lock, with the screw head adjacent to the grooved surface of the under finger guard.

Traction, with the head in the transverse position, will bring the head well down into the plane of the outlet before rotation is begun (Figs. 8–11, 8–12). Rotation is counterclockwise for a left occiput transverse (L.O.T.) presentation and clockwise for a right occiput transverse (R.O.T.), to the anterior position. The handles are rotated over a wide arc, using the center of the head as a pivot point (Figs. 8–13, 8–14). The handle of the traction attachment should remain in the midline during rotation. At the completion of rotation, the handles are parallel to or a little below the horizontal. They are directed obliquely away from the midline toward the opposite side. Thus, after rotation of an L.O.T. to anterior, the handles are near the patient's right thigh; after rotation of an R.O.T., the handles are near the left thigh (Figs. 8–15, 8–16).

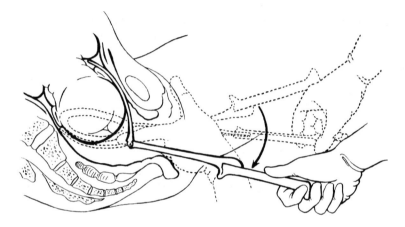

FIGURE 8–4. The hinged Barton blade has been "wandered" by the index and middle fingers of the *left* hand around the *right* side of the pelvis over the *occiput* of a *flexed* R.O.T. to the anterior, or left, ear behind the symphysis. The handle is held in the *right* hand. If this R.O.T. had been *extended*, the hinged instrument would have been held in the *left* hand and "wandered" by the fingers of the *right* hand, around the *left* side of the pelvis over the *face* to the anterior, or left, ear.

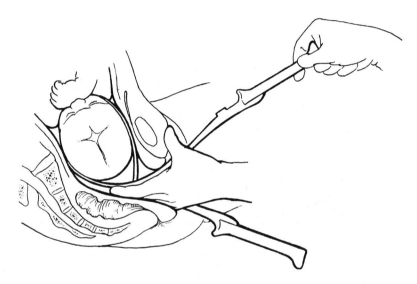

FIGURE 8–5. Introduction of posterior, rigid blade of Barton forceps, between the handle of the anterior, hinged blade and the right thigh, directly to the posterior left ear of L.O.T.

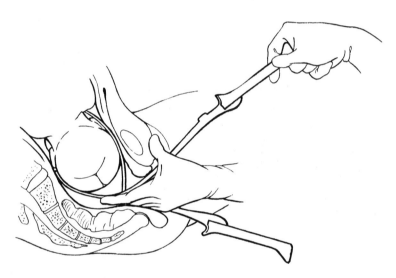

FIGURE 8–6. Introduction of posterior, rigid blade of Barton forceps between the handle of the anterior, hinged blade and the right thigh, directly to the posterior right ear of R.O.T.

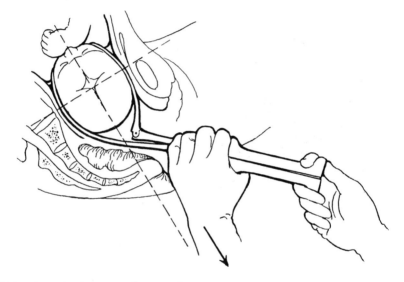

FIGURE 8–7. Application of Barton forceps to L.O.T. Any asynclitism had been corrected by equalizing the handles.

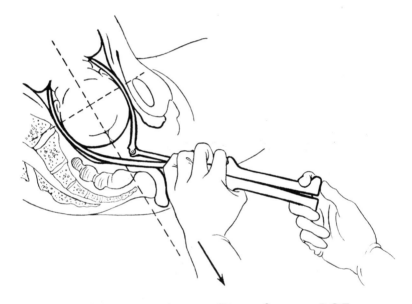

FIGURE 8–8. Application of Barton forceps to R.O.T.

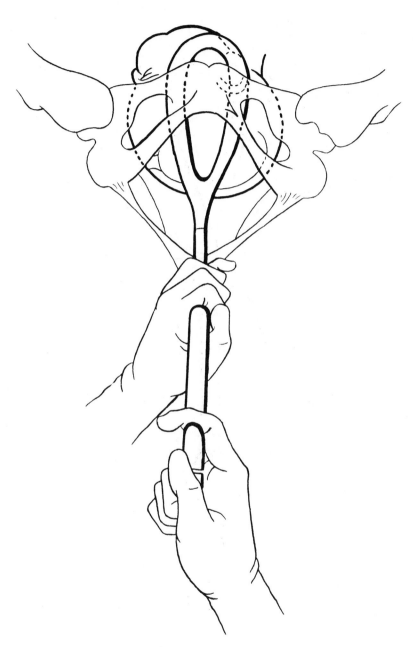

FIGURE 8–9. Front view of Barton forceps applied to L.O.T.

Forceps Deliveries

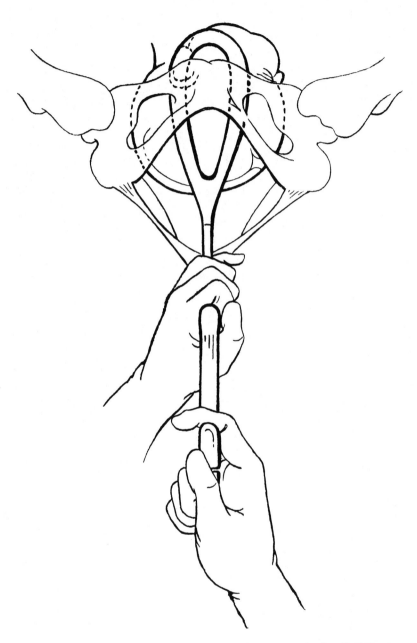

FIGURE 8–10. Front view of Barton forceps applied to R.O.T.

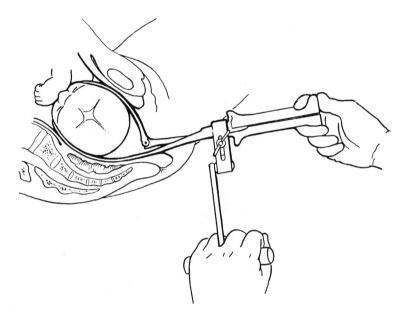

FIGURE 8–11. Barton forceps with axis-traction handle, ready for traction on L.O.T. Anterior rotation is not performed until the head is near the outlet.

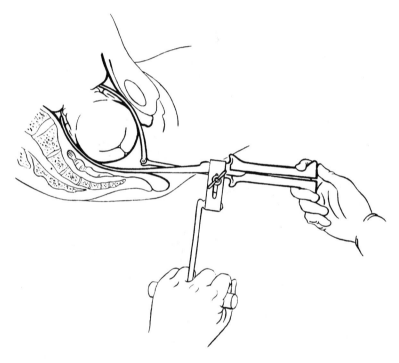

FIGURE 8–12. Barton forceps with axis-traction handle ready for traction on R.O.T. without anterior rotation until head is well down in the pelvis.

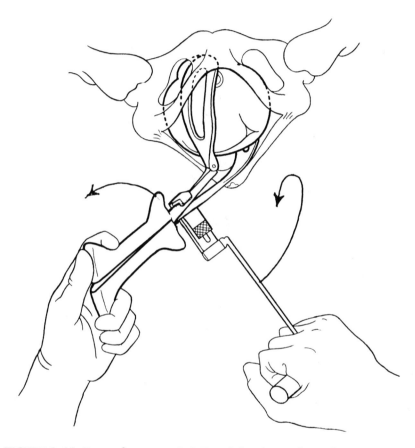

FIGURE 8–13. Barton forceps on L.O.T. with head near the outlet preparatory to counterclockwise rotation to O.A.

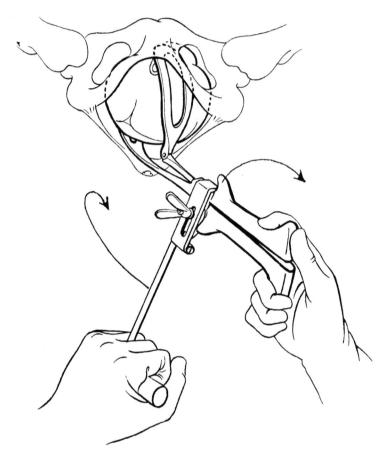

FIGURE 8–14. Barton forceps on R.O.T. with head near the outlet preparatory to clockwise rotation to O.A.

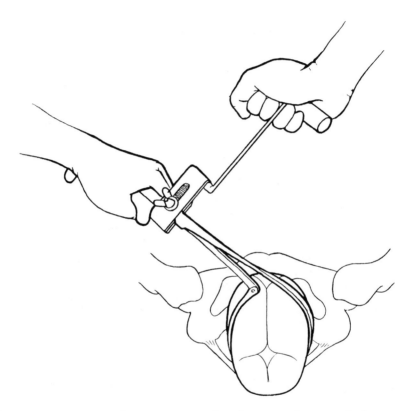

FIGURE 8–15. Barton forceps on O.A. after descent and counterclockwise rotation from L.O.T. to anterior, ready for traction and extension. The handles are directed away from the midline toward the right thigh.

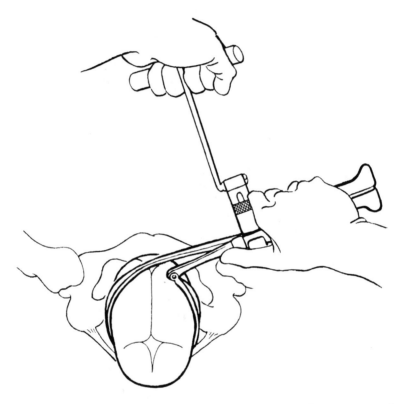

FIGURE 8–16. Barton forceps on O.A. after descent and clockwise rotation from R.O.T. to anterior, ready for traction and extension. The handles are directed away from the midline toward the left thigh.

Traction is applied by one hand in the direction of the shank of the axis traction handle. The other hand grasps the handles of the forceps to guide the direction of the force and to aid in extension during the traction. Extension is accomplished by continued pull with the traction handle in the midline, while all handles are elevated moderately above the horizontal. At a point where a Ritgen maneuver may be performed, the blades are removed and delivery is accomplished.

In a primipara, resistance to extension over the perineum may be encountered even after an episiotomy and lowering of the legs. This is due to the loss of the availability of the pelvic curve of the instrument after anterior rotation. In such a case, the Barton forceps is removed after descent and rotation have been accomplished, and a classical instrument is applied to complete the delivery.

The chief indication for the Barton forceps is the chief contraindication for the Kielland forceps, namely, transverse arrest with posterior parietal presentation, especially in the pelvis with short anteroposterior diameters. The necessary traction in the transverse diameter cannot be made with the Kielland instrument on this type of case, as in this position its pelvic curve and axis traction cannot be utilized. This is particularly true at mid pelvis or higher. In the presence of a straight sacrum shortening the anteroposterior diameter at mid pelvis, the risks are more pronounced. With the Barton forceps, it is possible to make traction to this position because, when applied, it has an excellent pelvic curve and good axis traction. The force, therefore, is in the axis of the pelvis away from the symphysis and the bladder. The head can be drawn well down in the transverse diameter, into the outlet, passing the point of obstruction before anterior rotation is done.

POSTERIOR POSITIONS

Although seen infrequently, posterior oblique positions can exist in which the Barton forceps may be indicated. As previously noted, this would be in instances of shortened anteroposterior diameters.

Left Occiput Posterior

In the left occiput posterior (L.O.P.) position, the hinged anterior blade is applied first, directly to the anterior ear, instead of by the wandering maneuver as in the transverse position. This is particularly true with a lower position of the head in the pelvis, which allows direct upward application. The blade is held in the left hand and is guided by two fingers of the right hand to the left anterior side of the pelvis just in front of the right, or anterior, ear. An assistant holds it in place. The handle of the posterior blade is held in the right hand and the toe is guided to the right posterior side of the pelvis, just in front of the left, or posterior, ear.

After locking and equalizing the handles and attaching the traction bar, counterclockwise rotation is performed over an arc to bring the occiput to transverse. Traction followed by rotation and extension maneuvers are then performed in the usual manner, as previously described.

Right Occiput Posterior

The technique of application to a right occiput posterior (R.O.P.) is similar to that of the L.O.P. except that the order of the sides is reversed. The hinged blade, held in the right hand, is inserted first, directly to the right anterior side of the pelvis opposite the left, or anterior, ear. The posterior blade, held in the left hand, is inserted directly to the left posterior side of the pelvis opposite the right, or posterior, ear. The rotation is clockwise to occiput transverse (O.T.), followed by the same maneuvers as for O.T. positions.

The best results with this instrument on posterior positions are obtained when the head is well down in the pelvis. If the head has to be brought down in the posterior oblique position before it can be rotated, the Barton forceps loses part of its good pelvic curve and good axis traction. Hence, incomplete rotation as far as the transverse position should be performed as soon as possible. Traction is continued in this position until the biparietal diameter has reached well below the level of the ischial spines before completing the rotation to the anterior position.

Again, the exceptions to this maneuver are android and anthropoid pelves. With a short transverse diameter of the pelvis, traction should be made on a head in the anteroposterior diameter. Under these conditions, the Kielland forceps is much more effective.

NINE

Special Instruments: Piper Forceps for the Aftercoming Head

The decision of whether or not to deliver a breech vaginally is not within the purview of this book. However, when vaginal delivery is elected, or in an emergency situation in which the breech is already partially delivered, the operator should consider forceps to the after-coming head.

A reduction of up to 50 percent in the morbidity of breech delivery has been ascribed to forceps use. The flexion attitude of the fetal head is strictly controlled by the forceps as the head is moved through the pelvis. There is no traction force on the trunk or cervical spine of the infant. Consequently, hyperextension injury is avoided. This is always a potential problem with a Mauriceau-Smellie-Veit maneuver that is other than very simple or when the head does not descend readily. Possible injury to the tentorium from suprapubic pressure on the skull is avoidable with forceps that apply force to the most resistant part, namely, the bimalar biparietal region. Delayed descent of the head subjects the infant to an increased hypoxia risk, avoidable with a timely, forceps-controlled descent. The less experienced operator can be expected to lose much of the dread of vaginal breech deliveries following preparatory training and routine use of forceps to the aftercoming head.

The Piper forceps was designed by Edmund B. Piper of Philadelphia, in 1924, for use on the aftercoming head of breech deliveries.

Construction

The long shanks have a backward curve, like a reverse pelvic curve, at about the middle. This drops the handles to a considerable distance below the level of the blades. The other chief difference in the shanks is the development of individual planes. The plane of the shanks is in the same plane as that of the blades to a point about 5 cm (2 inches) from the lock, whereas the lower 5 cm (2 inches) are in the plane of the handles. In the classical instrument, the plane of the shank is in the same plane as that of the handle throughout its entire length. This unique type of construction of the shanks in the Piper forceps gives more spring to the blades. With more spring to the blades, there tends to be less compression of the head. The blade is a modification of the Tarnier instrument, having a small cephalic and slight pelvic curve.

Advantages

The dropped handles allow a direct application to the sides of the head without elevating the body above the horizontal, thereby preventing injury to the fetal neck.

The spring of the blades, made possible by the long portion of the shanks lying in the same plane as the blades, causes less compression of the head.

The backward bend of the shanks gives axis traction.

Disadvantages

The blade has a straight pelvic curve and may cause some damage to the outlet during extension if an episiotomy is not performed. This is a minor consideration since the straight pelvic curve is necessary in order to make a direct application to a higher head. The spring in the blade along with the slender, almost straight, cephalic curve may cause slipping on a large round head or if the application is not accurate.

Technique

After the shoulders and arms have been delivered and the head is in the pelvis with the chin posterior, the Piper forceps should be applied. The position of the head is quickly verified by feeling for the chin with the examining finger. It usually is directly posterior or within a few degrees of posterior. The infant should be supported and the extremities removed from the field with the Savage maneuver, in which a towel sling for the infant is placed and held by the assistant. The assistant should be cautioned against the natural impulse to improve vision by elevating the infant above the horizontal. The left blade is applied first, in order to avoid difficulty in locking. The assistant carries the infant's body toward the mother's right side, staying horizontal. The body must never be extended over the symphysis unless the infant is "face to pubis." With the infant's body carried toward the right side, the approach to the left side of the pelvis is more direct and less difficult.

The operator assumes a kneeling or low sitting position in front of the patient. The left blade, held in the left hand, is inserted to the left side of the pelvis over the infant's right ear (the third exception to the cardinal point of left blade to the left ear for forceps application) (Fig. 9–1). If the head is in the anteroposterior diameter, the left blade goes directly to the side of the pelvis. If the head is in the left occiput anterior, or right oblique diameter, the left blade is the posterior blade. When the head is in the right occiput anterior, or left oblique diameter, the left blade is the anterior blade. In each instance, the left blade is applied first, directly to the side of the head. The handle of the forceps is held almost at right angles to the patient, below her right thigh and beneath the body of the infant, while the toe of the blade is guided into the vagina with two fingers of the right hand.

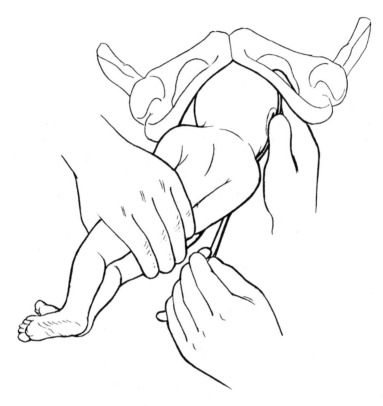

FIGURE 9–1. Insertion from below upward of first, or left, blade of the Piper forceps to the right ear of the aftercoming head.

The handle is swept in an arc downward and toward the midline, while the toe of the blade passes into the pelvis along the side of the infant's head to the right ear. The direction of the blade relative to the horizontal will vary with the station of the head, but generally should be close to 45 degrees below the horizontal. Experimentation on the manikin will show the operator that owing to its difference from a classical instrument, the toe of the blade can readily be directed into the pelvic wall or sacrum if the direction is incorrect. The assistant then carries the infant's body toward the patient's left thigh, exposing the approach to the right side of the pelvis. The right blade is similarly introduced by the right hand to the right side of the pelvis opposite the infant's left ear (Fig. 9–2). If resistance is met, the toe of the blade is introduced more posteriorly and wandered around to the side of the head. After the shanks have been locked, the infant is allowed to straddle the forceps. The handles rest in the upturned palm of the right hand with the middle finger in the space between the shanks.

After application of the forceps, if the head is not in a direct anterior position, it is rotated instrumentally, and downward traction is made from the kneeling or sitting position in the direction of the handles until the chin appears at the outlet. The handles are then elevated with traction in order to conform to the curve of the pelvis and to promote and preserve flexion during delivery of the head over the perineum. While making traction, the right thumb grasps the infant's thigh over the forceps handles, so that when the head is extracted, it will not fall through the blades. The index and middle fingers of the left hand press on the suboccipital region, splinting the neck and helping to bring the occiput under the arch (Fig. 9–3). If resistance is encountered at the outlet after an episiotomy has been performed, the handles of the blades are depressed and elevated during gentle traction in a pump-handle maneuver. This favors delivery of the head over the perineum with less effort and less injury; first, by bringing the suboccipital region further under the arch, and second, by increasing the flexion. Finally, extraction is performed with the handles close to the horizontal, delivering the head with the forceps still in place (Fig. 9–4).

The very rare "face-to-pubis" situation is usually avoided by the method of delivery of the body, shoulders, and arms. Should one

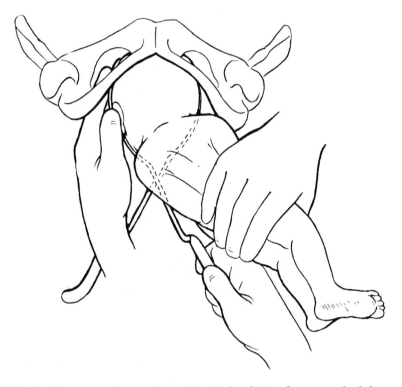

FIGURE 9–2. Insertion of second, or right, blade of Piper forceps to the left ear of aftercoming head.

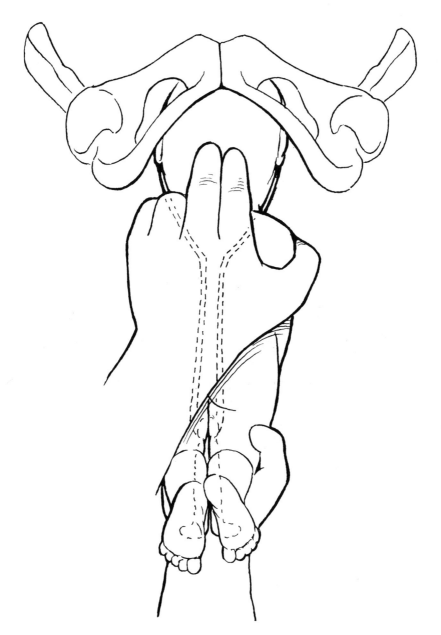

FIGURE 9–3. Piper forceps on aftercoming head during traction. Body resting on shanks, leg clamped to handle by thumb, handles resting in upturned palm of right hand with middle finger in the space between the shanks at the lock, neck splinted by fingers of the left hand.

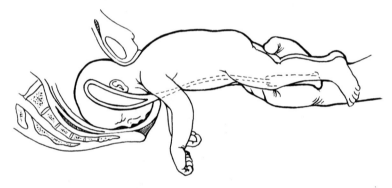

FIGURE 9–4. Application of Piper forceps to aftercoming head which is about to be delivered over perineum by flexion without removal of the forceps.

encounter a face-up aftercoming head, if a bimanual maneuver fails to deliver the aftercoming head, the forceps are applied. The approach is from below upward, under the infant's back, directly to the sides of the head, the leading point of which is now the occiput. Following traction, the occiput is delivered over the mother's perineum with the chin facing the pubis. Simultaneously, the legs and body are carried up over the symphysis.

A classical type of forceps may be used on the aftercoming head, but its disadvantages make it rather undesirable. The pelvic curve and the straight shanks require elevation of the infant's body toward the symphysis to permit application of the blades beneath it. This risks injury to the neck and tends to extend the head. The forward bend of the shanks and handles tends to interfere with complete instrumental flexion of the head. The rigid blades can give more compression to the head. Unless the instrument has such an attachment, axis traction cannot be utilized.

If the disadvantages of the Piper forceps in any individual case are apparent, there are alternatives that can be used to advantage. The Hawks-Dennen forceps, with similar principles of construction to the Piper, has less spring in the blades than the Piper plus an ample cephalic curve suitable for large heads. The reverse or backward pelvic curve and the sliding lock of the Kielland forceps favor a direct and accurate application and a good line of traction. Both the Hawks-Dennen and the Kielland forceps have been used successfully and are routinely preferred for the aftercoming head by some operators.

TEN

Special Instruments: Other

Special instruments that apply the axis traction principle are available. The importance of axis traction cannot be underestimated. As previously stated, to use the least force in accomplishing descent of the head, traction must be in the pelvic axis. Manual methods of axis traction, at any level of the pelvis, require an estimation of relative forces applied. This is essentially the obstetrician's subjective impression and is a potential for deviation from the optimal course. The possibility of trauma to fetus and mother is lessened by an instrument, or attachment, that decreases force wasted in the wrong direction. Also, the operator can more easily evaluate the amount of traction force actually applied to the head when the vectored force is supplied by an axis traction instrument and is a straight pull.

Bill Handle

The Bill axis traction handle has been mentioned several times previously. It is an important addition to our instruments in that it is a device that attaches to a classical instrument, resulting in automatic axis traction (Fig. 10–1).

The Bill handle has two shafts connected with a hinge. At the

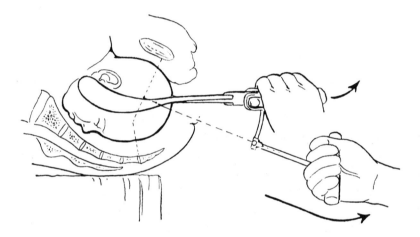

FIGURE 10–1. Instrumental axis traction. Tucker-McLane, solid blades with Bill handle.

hinge is a lateral marker that indicates the correct position of the hinge when in use. One shaft ends in hooks that slip over the finger guards of the previously applied forceps. The other shaft ends in the traction bar, which is dropped over the perineum, down into the long axis of the head. No vectoring of forces is necessary since tractive force on the handle is directly applied in the proper direction (assuming correct application has been performed). This greatly facilitates traction.

Hawks-Dennen Forceps

A light, fixed axis traction forceps, best suited to any anterior position of the head, was designed by E.M. Hawks and E.H. Dennen. The blades are a Simpson-type modification. The long cephalic curve has the tips lengthened with an exaggerated curve of the posterior lips. The fenestrated blades have beveled inner surfaces, decreasing the chance of bruising or cutting. The shanks are a modification of the Piper instrument, having a reverse pelvic curve in the middle, although shorter and with a sharper curve than the Piper. The curve in the shanks is such that the finger guards lie in the long axis of the head when the forceps are properly applied. This results in axis traction in all cases (Figs. 10–2, 10–3).

The instrument may be used as a primary tractor, or it may be used following rotation by another instrument, when a better traction device is desired. The longer cephalic curve fits molded heads evenly, and the toes seat well below the malar eminences. In positions other than occiput in an anterior quadrant, other instruments are preferable. Exceptions to this would be in the case of delivery as an occiput posterior, mentum anterior, or aftercoming head.

The technique of application is similar to that of the classical forceps. The operator must remember the reverse pelvic curve of the shanks. Prior to insertion, the handles must be held angled laterally away from the midline in order to adjust for the backward curve of the shanks. With insertion, the handle naturally drops to a lower level than with the classical instrument. Similarly, with extension, if the handles are elevated much over the horizontal, there is increased

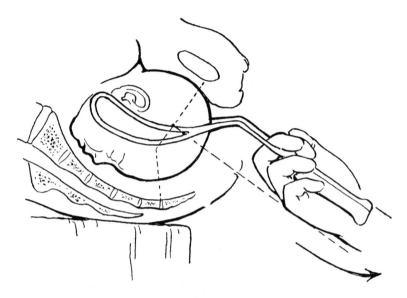

FIGURE 10–2. Instrumental axis traction. Hawks-Dennen.

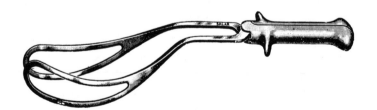

FIGURE 10–3. Hawks-Dennen forceps with perineal curve for axis traction.

risk of the toes injuring the sulci, despite the increased curve of the posterior lip of the blade. Slightly more room on the perineum is required owing to the space between the shanks at the heels of the blades, as is the case with any Simpson type of forceps.

DeWees Forceps

This instrument was more popular in the past, but it is still frequently available. Some operators claim to have observed an increased frequency of injuries associated with it. The general configuration of the instrument is a spread shank Simpson type. It has a French lock with a wing nut screw device to tighten the blades on the fetal skull. The traction bar is dropped by an extension attached to one handle so that axis traction is automatic (Fig. 10–4).

Other similar examples of a Simpson-type instrument with attachments for axis traction which may be available are the Lobstein-Tarnier and the Good. In addition to being cumbersome, these instruments were all designed for difficult higher-level forceps procedures that should probably be avoided.

Mann Forceps

The instrument developed by J. Mann in 1956 (not his earlier instrument) employs rigid blades and parallel shanks. The blades are connected with a wedge-shaped sliding lock. This device permits the blades to slide to different depths into the pelvis to adjust for asynclitism. The instrument is claimed to automatically adjust itself as the asynclitism disappears during rotation. Simultaneously, the shanks remain parallel while adjusting to heads of different sizes by locking at varying distances from each other. A bar attaches to the lock, serving as a handle for rotation and axis traction. The relatively straight pelvic curve permits application in any position of the occiput. Compression is minimized. Rotation and traction may be accomplished without reapplication of the instrument.

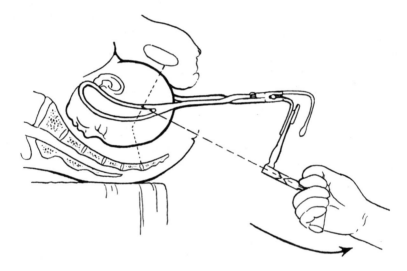

FIGURE 10–4. Instrumental axis traction. DeWees.

Miseo Forceps

Another attempt to develop the universal obstetrical forceps is the instrument reported by A. Miseo in 1956. This employs adjacent shanks to which the blades articulate at a split universal joint. The anterior blade is also hinged to allow application similar to that of the anterior blade of the Barton forceps. The hinge position and pressure to grasp the head can be adjusted with a turn knob in the handle. The ball-and-socket universal joint can be rotated in any plane or direction in the socket formed by the union of the proximal shanks. The joint can be locked and made rigid at any appropriate time. The thin blades are moderately fenestrated, and the pelvic curve has been eliminated from them.

The forceps can be applied in any position of the occiput, with application in the transverse aided by the hinged anterior blade. Compression is minimized. After rotation and during descent, the universal joint can be unlocked to permit the head to follow the path of least resistance while axis traction is applied. No reapplication should be necessary.

Laufe Forceps

The new obstetric forceps described by L. Laufe in 1956 ingeniously incorporates features of the Kielland and the Barton forceps, looking for the advantages of both in a single instrument. Superficially, there is a similarity to the Kielland instrument in length, handles, and sliding lock. The blade is longer and wider, but symmetrical, lacking the Kielland's slight reverse curve in the shanks. The shank on the handle without the lock is hinged behind the blade, allowing an application similar to that of the anterior blade of the Barton forceps. After application, the hinge can be locked at the shank, thus giving a rigid instrument.

The technique of application for transverse positions of the occiput is similar to that of the Barton forceps. The Kielland inversion technique for the anterior blade is never used with this instrument. For occiput posterior and other positions, the technique is the same as that of the Kielland forceps. Following application, rotation and extraction are performed as with the Kielland.

With each of the preceding three instruments described above (Mann, Miseo, and Laufe forceps), availability and popularity willl vary in different areas of the country. When considering clever designs that strive for the universal forceps, it must be remembered that as one advantage is gained, another is often lost. In elimination of certain classical instrument features, which are disadvantages under certain conditions but are advantages under others, new disadvantages are often created. This is particularly true in more complicated cases. Other problems encountered in instruments with multiple moving parts are cleaning and maintenance.

Other instruments, such as the Leff forceps and the Shute forceps, of ingenious, inventive, and thoughtful design, have appeared. Perhaps undeservedly, they have not attracted wide acceptance and distribution.

Divergent Forceps

An unusual instrument is the divergent outlet forceps as introduced by L. Laufe in 1968. Although others of similar concept are available, this is the most popular for outlet use.

The shanks are of the Elliot type, and the blades have a Luikart type of indented fenestration. There is a perineal curve without a pronounced pelvic curve. The blades are joined by a pivot lock at the end of the shanks. There are no handles; instead, finger grips for traction are present, each located on the same side of the lock as its respective blade. Since no crossed first class lever exists, compression of the fetal head by force transmitted from handle compression is not possible. Traction on the finger grips applies negative (divergent) force on the skull, due to the physics of this arrangement. This somewhat reduces compression of the head.

The instrument is maintained in its position on the fetal head during traction by the compressive force of pressure from the maternal pelvis and soft parts.

Vectis

One blade of a forceps, or a special instrument, may be used as a vectis to assist in delivery of the head through the uterine incision at cesarean section. The operator's hand cupped beneath the head and aiding extraction greatly increases the necessary circumference of the uterine incision. Extensions of the incision are not uncommon, may be difficult to repair, and involve extra blood loss.

A vectis aids rotation and elevation of the head and helps to deliver the head by extension, as with vaginal delivery. It can act similarly to an inclined plane directing the head when fundal pressure is applied. It occupies very little space, and extensions of the incision are rare.

Although a single forceps blade may be used, the type of vectis that is symmetrical, having only a fenestrated cephalic curve on a shank and handle, is easier to use. The operator inserts one hand in the uterine incision, feeling the direction of the sagittal suture, as the toe of the vectis is inserted. It is moved between the fingers and the head, usually over the parietal bone. With the hand removed, the vectis is lifted and turned to direct the occiput upward and through the incision, propelled by fundal pressure.

The use of a special, short Simpson-type forceps and even the vacuum extractor has also been advocated for extraction of the head at cesarean section. These are felt to be more cumbersome and time consuming. It is always advisable to deliver the fetal head in as short a time as possible following the uterine incision.

Vacuum Extractor

Although the use of the vacuum extractor (VE) is not really within the scope of a book on forceps deliveries, it must be considered as a possible forceps alternative.

Descriptions of the VE history, instrumentation, and technique are available elsewhere. In some European countries, the VE is currently the predominant method of instrumental delivery when indicated for fetal distress or poor second stage of labor. In the United States, some enthusiasm for the instrument was seen following its introduction, but its acceptance has generally been much more limited. This is quite possibly related to the scalp effects, since the method, almost by definition, involves universal scalp trauma.

Although Malmström originally described application of the VE to a scalp prior to full dilatation of the cervix and at *any* station of the head, the reported subsequent higher incidence of fetal injury has altered the indications. Currently, use at high station and with incomplete cervical dilatation is discouraged. Extended length of traction, prolonged usage, and active rotation are similarly predisposing to more severe injuries. It does appear that careful use, in appropriate cases, by an experienced operator is safe. As with forceps procedures, assessment of indications plus fetal and maternal factors is mandatory prior to application.

Several advantages of the instrument are reported. Less anesthesia is required. It has a wide margin of safety for the mother, with decreased risk of maternal lacerations. In selected cases, earlier and more active intervention is possible in cases of fetal distress, since it is often reportedly used at +1 station or higher, where forceps use is contraindicated. The size of the head is not increased by the addition of instrumentation. Some deviations from the normals of position and attitude can be corrected, depending on the site of application of the VE. The method can easily be abandoned for another modality in case of failure.

The main disadvantages relate to the fetal effects of the instrument. The artificial caput succedaneum appearance is distasteful, but is only cosmetic and usually disappears in several days. The more severe sequelae of scalp trauma, including abrasion, laceration, or even avulsion of the scalp, may occur. Similarly, ecchymosis, sub galeal hemorrhage, cephalhematoma, and retinal hemorrhage have been reported. The potential for intracranial injury exists; tentorial tears and intracranial hemorrhage have been seen. The possibility of injury constitutes a relative contraindication in the premature infant, and caution is advised following scalp puncture for pH determination. The incidence of neonatal jaundice is increased. There is an appreciable method failure rate due to slippage and a limitation of the amount of traction that can safely be applied. A certain amount of time is required to establish the vacuum. The control of the head is less than with forceps delivery.

Reports on the newer Silastic Obstetrical Vacuum Cup indicate that a reduction of the scalp sequelae without appreciable loss of effectiveness of the technique may be possible with that instrument.

It is obviously difficult for a forceps protagonist to view the vacuum extractor with complete objectivity. Most authors, including VE advocates, agree that forceps deliveries can be only partially replaced by this instrument. Certainly, the method is probably not advisable as an elective procedure in view of the cosmetic problem to the infant. There appears to be a potential use for it in transverse and posterior arrests, although these are the cases in which the highest incidence of method failure may be anticipated. The protracted second stage of labor and fetal distress may also be indications, depending on the individual circumstances, not the least of which would be the experience and skill of the operator.

ELEVEN

Choices—Conclusion

An early choice on the part of the obstetrician is that of elective or prophylactic forceps. Despite the often strident consumer cries that natural is better, compelling evidence collected over the past several decades strongly suggests improved short- and long-term fetal results with outlet forceps rather than spontaneous delivery. On the other hand, the practicing physician, mindful of the realities of the marketplace, is usually reluctant to voice this opinion. The author, in spite of a firmly held belief in elective forceps, has no set personal policy other than prudent patient education (even during labor or after delivery) and would not presume to advise the reader on the best course of action in this respect. Certainly, the procedure can be expected to do no harm, while potentially providing fetal and maternal benefits.

When the obstetrician is presented with a situation in which a fetal or maternal indication for intervention with the course of a labor exists, many choices arise. The variables in a clinical situation are essentially limitless. They must be evaluated, however, in an effort to decide the most appropriate action within the given circumstances.

All of the prerequisites for forceps delivery must be considered. The patient, her pelvis, and her labor pattern should be evaluated. A fetal status assessment that includes general condition, estimation of size, and determination of position, attitude, station, and degree of molding should be made. The available facilities, services, and support staff are also important. Finally, the operator's knowledge of the instruments, as well as his or her personal skill and limitations, should be weighed in the choices.

The initial choice is the general course of action, namely, abdominal delivery, vaginal forceps delivery, trial of forceps, or vacuum extractor. Next, the choice of instrument must be made. Lastly, during performance of the procedure, choices of technique become necessary.

As has previously been stated, the elective and low forceps procedures have been shown to give results at least equivalent to spontaneous vaginal delivery. Mid forceps procedures have fetal results comparable to cesarean section, particularly when the procedures are performed for similar indications. There is general agreement on the advantage of the "easy" mid forceps delivery. A considerable problem exists in the prospective determination of which case should be easy. With a problem case, collection and consideration of all the available clinical information should result in a greatly decreased incidence of the unanticipated difficult mid forceps that, in retrospect, should have been avoided. Certainly, if one is not reasonably certain, there is reason for cautious trial forceps (or *"trial of forceps"*).

It has long been the strong belief of the author that there is a definite place for the trial of forceps. In this respect, the use of the term "failed forceps" is not advised. That specific negative term can stigmatize by implying that the procedure was abandoned after repeated attempts proved it to be impossible. Historically, "failed forceps" has suggested judgmental error and bad obstetrics, possibly negligence. A "trial of forceps," on the other hand, connotes a tentative attempt at a forceps delivery with the reservation to alter treatment if potentially dangerous resistance or difficulty is met. Performed with care and caution, usually with a double setup, or as preparations are being made for cesarean section, it can prove fruitful and safe.

A forceps trial is *not* indicated for inlet dystocia or other problems at the inlet. Conditions such as a known pelvic abnormality with apparent feto-pelvic disproportion, the brow presentation, the chin posterior face presentation, many previously diagnosed fetal anomalies, and the dead fetus with postmortem changes should not be considered for a trial of forceps, for obvious reasons. Indications for a trial of forceps should be critically considered in the case of labor arrests with the vertex at mid pelvic level (i.e., biparietal at plane of greatest pelvic dimensions, hollow of the sacrum not filled). An appreciably higher incidence of depressed infants, shoulder dystocia, and maternal trauma can result. Protraction disorders treated by mid forceps intervention are stated to be associated with an increased incidence of perinatal mortality. The procedure in such cases should be assessed with proper gravity.

In appropriate circumstances and with the availability of abdominal delivery in case of negative results, the trial of forceps is a valuable and eminently acceptable procedure. After evaluation of all available data, a gentle and judicious trial at low or mid forceps level may be carried out. A careful attempt at application, rotation as necessary, and traction do not injure an infant. Injury is the result of force applied to tissues that resist that force, regardless of reason. That resistance can be felt and is quite obvious. If the operator refuses to apply force of injurious quantity, injury cannot occur.

In the case of the premature and low-birth-weight infant, forceps were believed, in the past, to provide protection from trauma and its potential neurologic sequelae. Some recent studies have demonstrated cesarean section to be preferable when estimated fetal weight is in the very-low-birth-weight range (below 1500 grams) or when the presentation is other than vertex. Estimation of fetal weight can become critical to proper management strategy, and ultrasound evaluation should be used, despite the possible (< 10 percent) error rate. In the over-1500-gram infant, whether premature or small for gestational age, the cesarean section advantage is not present. In this group, no significant difference is reported between spontaneous and low forceps delivery, and cases should be individualized. It appears that fetal head compression is not a major determinant of intraventricular hemorrhage. There is a growing body of evidence that, in most instances, modern delivery methods have little relationship to infant outcome. Considerably more important are other factors that may contribute to neonatal depression and the skill of the perinatal management. Close collaboration between the obstetrician and the neonatologist is essential to improved results. The choice of delivery site must be made as well, depending on the availability of neonatal intensive care.

Choice of Instrument

Given a proper case for delivery with forceps, an operator must choose the kind of instrument most suitable for the conditions. Delivery may be accomplished with only one, or at most two varieties of forceps. However, other things being equal, a greater degree of success should be obtained with a knowledge of the advantages and a discrimination in the use of the various kinds of forceps. There are several kinds of forceps, old and new, that have peculiar advantages under certain conditions. The unique clinical advantages of each instrument are lost if one attempts to do everything with a single forceps.

In delivery with forceps under proper conditions, there are two features of prime importance. First is the application of the forceps to the fetal head. Secondly, assuming that rotation of 45 degrees or less is required, is the traction used in accomplishing the delivery. These two acts determine the manipulation and effort required and, consequently, the associated trauma.

In a proper cephalic application, the blades should fit the head as accurately as possible. They should lie evenly against the sides of the head, reaching from the parietal bosses to, and beyond, the malar eminences, symmetrically covering the spaces between the orbits and the ears. There should be no extra pressure at any one point, so that pressure is evenly distributed and directed to the least vulnerable areas.

In the choice of an instrument with which a good application can be obtained, much depends on a correct diagnosis of the amount of molding, the position, station, and attitude of the head, and the type of pelvis.

On molded heads, the best application is obtained with blades that have a long, tapering, cephalic curve. Those with a short, full curve do not fit evenly, causing pressure points, and often they are not anchored below the malar eminences, with consequent cutting or slipping. In considering the position of the head, the instrument to be chosen is the one that gives the correct application with the least effort. When the occiput is anterior, the application is, as a rule, easily made, and any blade that fulfills the requirements of the molding may be used. For other positions and presentations, there are special types to be considered with the various forceps operations. A head in the upper part of a flat pelvis or in a pelvis with a straight sacrum may be angulated in such a position that a cephalic application cannot be obtained unless the forceps has a flexible blade.

Traction also plays a very important part in the choice of the forceps. To use the least force, traction must be in the pelvic axis. This may be done manually, but it is best accomplished in all stations of the head with some form of axis traction forceps. Even in outlet forceps, axis traction is helpful in eliminating wasted force. To some, axis traction suggests a difficult operation with a complicated instrument. For this reason, it is often neglected in the average case, although the advantages are admitted. The classical forceps, without axis traction, are frequently used with the maximum force, aided by the Pajot or Saxtorph maneuver. Axis traction forceps, however, tend to keep the force in the plane of least resistance, thereby diminishing the amount of total effort required, as well as the injury potential.

In the selection of an instrument that fulfills the requirements of application and traction, there are many excellent forceps from which to choose. Some are simple; others complicated. All have one or more good points that justify their use when properly chosen. Some are so similar that there is very little choice between them. Various localities tend to have their favorites. Most modern forceps of the classical type generally follow one of two constructions: the shanks overlap and the blades have a short, cephalic curve as in the Elliot; or the shanks are separated and the blades have a long, tapering curve as in the Simpson. But not all of them have axis traction. This disadvantage can be overcome in some by the use of the Bill axis traction handle.

For easy extractions from outlet or low level, the thin solid blades of the Tucker-McLane (Elliot type) are popular with some obstetricians. They tend to fit best on small, rounder, less molded heads. They are easy to apply and remove but may slip owing to lack of anchorage below the malar eminences. In molded heads, they may exert pressure on two points: the zygoma and the parietal boss. The result may be a cut just in front of the ear, or the later appearance of a localized parietal periostitis. The Luikart modification, with an indented fenestration on the inner surface of the solid blade, minimizes this disadvantage and is favored by many for elective forceps. On occasion, what is thought to be an easy outlet forceps later proves to be a molded head in which the biparietal diameter is at or above the ischial spines. The operator then wishes that a fenestrated blade had originally been chosen.

The majority of cases requiring delivery by forceps are primiparous or multiparous with a prolonged labor, and more molding should be anticipated. With increased molding of the head, the separated shanks and longer, tapered cephalic curve of the Simpson-type forceps make that the preferred instrument. The toes of the blades can seat well below the malar eminences, preventing pressure points and slipping. The Hawks-Dennen forceps, an uncomplicated, light, fixed axis traction instrument with modified Simpson blades, can be chosen for any anterior position of the occiput at any station. Its advantages in application and traction tend to make the delivery easier and safer (see Chapter 10).

In the low and mid forceps operations, more frequently than in the outlet, the position, as well as the shape of the head, must be considered in the choice of a suitable type of instrument. The rules for anterior positions are the same in all stations of the head, with emphasis on axis traction. The Hawks-Dennen and DeWees forceps give excellent fixed axis traction and are considered the choice by some. With the head in transverse arrest, some operators have developed skill in the use of manual rotation or the wandering maneuver with a classical instrument. It is not an uncommon experience to find a head that cannot be rotated manually without displacement, or one that refuses to remain anterior during the process of applying the second blade and locking the handles. In the wandering maneuver, the anterior blade occasionally hits the brow, causing the occiput to rotate backward. This may result in a brow-mastoid application, which no amount of manipulation will entirely correct. To simplify this procedure, two special types of forceps are available, the Kielland and the Barton. Their chief advantage is the ease with which an accurate cephalic application can be obtained. Both have the sliding lock principle, which allows for adjustment on asynclitic heads. The Kielland, since it is a better tractor, has a wider field of usefulness and appears to be the choice, except in pelves with a straight sacrum or shortened anteroposterior diameters. However, the Barton, though less effective as a tractor, often requiring another type to complete the delivery, is chosen by some because its technique of application is simpler, or when the Kielland is contraindicated.

As previously noted under other special instruments, several other instruments may be available that may supply the advantages of single application for attitude correction, rotation, and traction from transverse as well as posterior positions.

In posterior positions, the single accurate application without displacement of the head, and semi axis traction pull after rotation with the Kielland forceps, involve less manipulation than the Scanzoni maneuver or manual rotation. The upside-down, direct application of the Kielland to an occiput posterior head permits rotation and extraction without readjustment of the blades. Exceptions to the procedure would be a marked anthropoid or android pelvis in which, because of limited space, it is considered necessary to deliver the posterior occiput, as such, without anterior rotation. Here, a Simpson type with axis traction is preferable in order to satisfy the requirements for molding and for the need of an instrument with a good pelvic curve and better traction. Should a Scanzoni maneuver be chosen, the solid blade Elliot-type instrument is preferred as a rotator in the first stage of the procedure.

Conclusion

The obstetrician is currently confronted by increasing demands from outside as well as within the profession, causing the specialty to be even more demanding than in the past. Forceps delivery, previously considered the hallmark of the obstetrician, is a valuable and necessary skill that should be taught and available as a management strategy alternative for all deliveries. The decrease in forceps learning experiences, whether due to program director decree or to consumer pressure, results in inexperienced operators whose only safe option in a difficult situation is abdominal delivery. This raises maternal cost, risks, and sequelae without improvement of fetal results.

Outlet and low forceps procedures, including elective forceps, have been demonstrated to have at least as good results as those obtained with spontaneous delivery. The same is true of mid forceps contrasted to cesarean section. Thus, the object of forceps delivery does not connote a "trade-off" of fetal versus maternal injury.

Observation of the prerequisites for forceps delivery is mandatory. The more obvious ruptured membranes, engaged head, fully dilated and retracted cervix, and appropriate anesthesia, equipment, and support personnel need no further comment. A working knowledge of obstetrical pelvic architecture is necessary to predict labor events and plan management. The initial pelvic examination during labor should include a clinical pelvimetry, checking information gained during the patient's prenatal course. A recheck of the pelvis after delivery, particularly with conduction anesthesia, is excellent for self-instruction. This can also be done from the opposite direction at cesarean section.

Since accurate application is so extremely important to safe forceps control of the fetal head, the intrapartum observations of position, attitude, and station assume greater import. If landmarks are obscured, the direction of the sagittal suture can at least be identified. (Example: sagittal suture in left oblique, running from right anterior to left posterior quadrant.) The information can be significant to the later course in labor, as can the observation of the fetal attitude of flexion or extension. Diagnosis of asynclitism and of the level of the biparietal diameter, and evaluation of labor for abnormalities of dilatation or descent, are equally significant prerequisites to forceps use. These factors should be looked for and recorded.

Proper traction, minimizing compression, is essential. Rotation to occiput anterior is usual and accomplished by manual, instrumental, or a combination method prior to traction. Traction must be in the axis of the pelvis to minimize necessary force and injury potential. Traction direction is critical, being properly applied perpendicular to the plane of the pelvis at the level of the biparietal diameter. Traction force must be controlled and carefully applied since force is required for injury and the objective is an atraumatic delivery.

The operator's knowledge of the instruments and choice of forceps to fit the individual case is certainly not the least of the prerequisites. The author disagrees with the concept of learning one instrument well so that everything may be accomplished with it. Most experienced operators have had cases in which delivery was too difficult with one instrument, but was completed successfully with another. It rarely takes more than one such experience to convince one that there is indeed a choice of forceps to suit the case.

Any intelligent operator with ordinary obstetrical skills can perform outlet, low, and even mid forceps procedures. With observance of the prerequisites and a cautious, gentle approach, most procedures are almost surprisingly simple when properly performed. The operator must think in a few terms with which he or she may be unfamiliar. First, think biparietal diameter: the measurement of the head that must be moved through the pelvis. It contains the pivot point of the head and is on the long axis of the head. Second, think the axis of the pelvis, to which traction should be perpendicular, and the long axis of the head, parallel. Third, think toes of the forceps blade rather than handles, since the toes must remain as close to the center of the pelvis as possible. Lastly, think plane of least resistance with application, rotation, and traction.

The operator must be prepared to abandon an unusually difficult procedure, evaluating reasons for the difficulty, trying a different approach, even allowing further labor or moving to abdominal delivery. The use of increased force is not an acceptable alternative. It is difficult to cause injury if one takes the force out of forceps.

Following all forceps deliveries, it is advisable to examine the infant for marks or signs of trauma. With the majority of procedures, little if any marking should be visible. When marks are visible, the symmetry and location should reassure the operator as to the correctness of application and traction. Variations from optimal technique will often be visible for several hours and can serve as a valuable learning tool. For example, if the forceps are not directed far enough below the horizontal in an oblique or transverse position, extra pressure on the anterior cheek will mark that cheek.

Concerning the medical-legal problem, the physician is advised to explain and to document all circumstances of the forceps delivery. An estimate of the degree of difficulty of the procedure should be recorded. As much laboratory support as possible should be used. In view of the currently prevailing patient prejudice concerning obstetrical forceps, patient education is indicated, certainly postpartum, if not antepartum or intrapartum. In this respect, an innocent past history question, "Was your delivery normal or by forceps?", can be prejudicial and potentially dangerous. For similar reasons, the frivolous term, "the hooks," is ill advised.

Studies related to forceps have been confusing and notoriously difficult to compare in the past. Opposite conclusions have been reported from presumably similar procedures by different investigators. At least part of the confusion has been due to a previously inadequate classification, a situation which should now be corrected. We are certain that forceps deliveries will continue to occupy a major place in the practice of obstetrics, important in the armamentarium lucinae.

Bibliography

Barton, LG, Caldwell, WE, and Studdiford, WE, Sr: A new obstetric forceps. Am J Obst & Gynec 15:16, 1928.

Behrman, SJ: Fetal cervical hyperextension. Clin Obst & Gynec 5:1018–1030, 1962.

Benedetti, TJ and Gabbe, SG: Shoulder dystocia: Complication of fetal macrosomia and prolonged second stage of labor with midpelvic delivery. Obstet Gynecol 52:526–529, 1978.

Bergman, P and Malmström, T: Natal and postnatal fetal mortality in association with vacuum extraction and forceps delivery. Gynaecologia 154:65–72, 1962.

Berkus, MD, Ramamurthy, RS, O'Connor, PS, Brown, K, and Hyashi, RH: Cohort studies of Silastic Obstetric Vacuum Cup deliveries: Safety of the instrument. Obstet Gynecol 66:503, 1985.

Bishop, EH, Israel, SL, and Briscoe, CL: Obstetrical influences on the premature infant's first year of development: A report from the Collaborative Study of Cerebral Palsy. Obstet Gynecol 26:628, 1965.

Bowes, WA and Bowes, C: Current role of the midforceps operation. Clin Obst & Gynec Vol. 23, No. 2, June 1980, Harper & Row.

Bowes, WA: Delivery of the very low birth weight infant. Clin Perinatol 8:18, 1981.

Broekhuizen, FF, Washington, J, Johnson, F, and Hamilton, PR: Vacuum extraction versus forceps deliveries: Indications and complications 1979 to 1984. Obstet Gynecol 69:338, 1987.

Cardoza, LD, Gibb, MF, Studd, JWW, and Cooper, DJ: Should we abandon Kielland's forceps? Br Med J 287, 315–317, 1983.

Cohen, W: Influence of the duration of second stage labor on perinatal outcome and puerperal morbidity. Obstet Gynecol 49:266–269, 1977.

Danforth, DN and Ellis, A: Mid forceps delivery: A vanishing art? Am J Obst & Gynec 86:29, 1963.

Danforth, DN: Midforceps delivery in the 1980's. Mediguide to Ob/Gyn Vol. 5, Issue 1.

Decker, W and Heaton, C: Barton Obstetric Forceps: An analysis of 277 cases. Am J Obst & Gynec 61:635, 1951.

DeLee, JB: Principles and Practice of Obstetrics, ed 6. 1934, WB Saunders.

Dennen, EH: Manual of forceps deliveries, privately printed, 1947.

Dennen, EH: Choice of instruments in delivery with forceps. New York State J Med 32:802, 1932.

Dennen, EH: A classification of forceps operations according to station of head in pelvis. Including results in 3,883 forceps deliveries. Am J Obst & Gynec 63:272, 1952.

Dennen, EH: The selection of an obstetric forceps to suit the case. Virginia Med Monthly 74:150, 1947.

Dennen, EH: Forceps Deliveries. 1964, FA Davis.

Dennen, EH: Techniques of application for low forceps. Clin Obst & Gynec 8:834, 1965.

Dieckmann, WJ: The place of operative obstetrics. Am J Obst & Gynec 69:1005, 1955.

Dierker, LJ, Rosen, MG, Thompson, RT, Linn, P, and Debanne, S: The midforceps: Maternal and neonatal outcomes. Am J Obst & Gynec 152:176, 1985.

Dierker, LJ, Rosen, MG, and Thompson, K: Midforceps deliveries: Long-term outcome of infants. Am J Obstet Gynec 154:764–768, 1986.

Douglas & Stromme Operative Obstetrics, ed 4. Appleton-Century-Crofts.

Duff, P: Diagnosis and management of face presentation. Obstet Gynecol 57:105, 1981.

Dyack, C: Rotational forceps in midforceps delivery. Obstet Gynecol 56:123–126, 1980.

Dyer, I: Trial and failed forceps. Clin Obst & Gynec 8:914, 1965.

Fairweather, D: Obstetric management of the very low birth weight infant. Jour Reprod Med 26:387–392, 1981.

Fall, O, Ryden, G, Finnstrom, K, Finnstrom, O, and Leijon, I: Forceps or vacuum extraction? A comparison of effects on the newborn infant. Acta Obstet Gynecol Scand 65:75–80, 1986.

Friedman, EA, Sachtleben, MR, and Bresky, PA: Dysfunctional labor: XII. Long-term effects on infant. Am J Obst & Gynec 127:779, 1977.

Friedman, EA, Sachtleben-Murray, MR, Dahrogue, D, and Neff, RK: Long-term effects of labor and delivery on offspring: A matched-pair analysis. Am J Obst & Gynec 50:941, 1984.

Friedman, E and Neff, RK: Labor & Delivery: Impact on offspring. 1987, PSG Publishing.

Gilstrap, LE, Hauth, JC, Schiano, S, and Connor, KD: Neonatal acidosis and method of delivery. Obstet Gynecol 63:681, 1984.

Gomez, HE and Dennen, EH: Face presentation: A study of 45 consecutive cases. Obstet Gynecol 8:103, 1956.

Healy, DL, Quinn, MA, and Pepperal, RJ: Rotational delivery of the fetus: Kielland's forceps and two other methods compared. Br J Obstet Gynaecol 89:501–506, 1982.

Healy, DL and Laufe, LE: Survey of obstetric forceps training in North America in 1981. Am J Obst & Gynec 151:54, 1985.

Hughey, MJ, McElin, TW, and Lussky, R: Forceps operations in perspective: I. Midforceps rotation operations. Jour Reprod Med 20:253–259, 1978. II. Failed operations. Jour Reprod Med 21:177–180, 1978.

Ingardia, CJ and Cetrulo, CL: Forceps: Use and abuse. Clinics in Perinatol 8:63, 1981.

Jarcho, J: The Kielland obstetrical forceps and its application. Am J Obst & Gynec 10:35, 1925.

Jewett, JF: Personal communications. 1983.

Kadar, N and Romero, R: Prognosis for future childbearing after midcavity instrumental deliveries in primigravidas. Obstet Gynecol 62:166, 1983.

Kielland, C: Direct personal communication and instruction. 1931 and 1937.

King, EL, Herring, JS, Dyer, I, and King, JA: The modification of the Scanzoni rotation in management of persistent occipitoposterior positions. Am J Obst & Gynec 61:872, 1951.

Laube, DW: Forceps Delivery. Clin Obst & Gynec Vol. 29, No. 2, 1986.

Laufe, LE: Obstetric Forceps. New York, Hoeber Medical Division of Harper & Row, 1968.

Luikart, R: A modification of the Kielland, Simpson, and Tucker-McLane forceps to simplify their use and improve function and safety. Am J Obst & Gynec 34:686, 1937.

Luikart, R: Methods for improving the results of forceps deliveries. J Obst & Gynaec (Brit Emp) 64:351, 1957.

Malmström, T: Vacuum Extractor: Indications and results. Acta Obst et Gynec Scandinav 43 (suppl 1):5–52, 1964.

Mann, J: Methods for improving the results of forceps delivery. J Obst & Gynaec (Brit Emp) Vol. 64, No. 3, 1957.

Milner, RDG: Neonatal mortality of breech deliveries with and without forceps to the aftercoming head. Br J Obstet Gynaecol 82:783–5, 1975.

Miseo, A: New obstetric forceps with a split universal joint principle. Obst & Gynec 8:487, 1956.

Moore, EJT and Dennen, EH: Management of persistent brow presentations. Obstet & Gynecol 6:186 (Aug) 1955.

Niswander, K and Gordon, M: The Collaborative Perinatal Study of the National Institute of Neurological Diseases and Stroke: The Women and their Pregnancies. Philadelphia, 1972, WB Saunders.

Niswander, K and Gordon, M: Safety of the low-forceps operation. Am J Obst & Gynecol 117:619–627, 1973.

Nyirjesy, I and Pierce, WE: Perinatal mortality and maternal morbidity in spontaneous and forceps vaginal deliveries. Am J Obst & Gynec 89:568–578, 1964.

O'Driscoll, K, Meagher, D, MacDonald, D, and Geoghagan, F: Traumatic intracranial haemorrhage in firstborn infants and delivery with obstetric forceps. Br J Obstet Gynaecol 88:577–581, 1981.

Pearse, WH: Electronic recording of forceps delivery. Am J Obst & Gynec 86:43, 1963.

Pelosi, MA and Apuzzio, J: Use of the soft silicone obstetric vacuum cup for delivery of the fetal head at cesarean section. Jour Reprod Med 19:289–292, 1984.

Pieri, RJ: The occipitoposterior position and the modified Scanzoni maneuver. New York State J Med 40:1773, 1940.

Piper, EB and Bachman, C: The prevention of fetal injuries in breech delivery. JAMA 92:217–221, 1929.

Plauche, WC: Fetal cranial injuries related to delivery with the Malmström vacuum extractor. Obstet Gynecol 53:750, 1979.

Posner, AC and Cohn, S: An analysis of forty five face presentations. Am J Obst & Gynec 62:592, 1951.

Pritchard, JR, MacDonald, PC, Gant, NF (eds): Williams Obstetrics, ed 17. New York, Appleton-Century-Crofts, 1985.

Reid, DE: A Textbook of Obstetrics. Philadelphia, WB Saunders, 1962.

Reiles, M and Pundel, FP: Application of forceps under local anesthesia. Gynec & Obst 61:414–422, 1962.

Richardson, DA, Evans, MI, and Cibils, LA: Midforceps delivery: A critical review. Am J Obst & Gynec 145:621, 1983.

Schwartz, DB, Miodovnik, M, and Lavin, JP: Neonatal outcome among low birth weight infants delivered spontaneously or by low forceps. Obstet Gynecol 62:283, 1983.

Smith, EC: New obstetric forceps for rotation and extraction of the fetal head in a single application. Am J Obst & Gynec 94:931–935, 1966.

Tejani, N, Verma, U, Hameed, C, and Chayen, B: Method and route of delivery in the low birth weight vertex presentation correlated with early periventricular/intraventricular hemorrhage. Obstet Gynecol 69:1, 1987.

Traub, AI, Morrow, RJ, Ritchie, JWK, and Dornan, KJ: A continuing use for Kielland's forceps? Br J Obstet Gynaecol 91:894–898, 1984.

Ullery, JC, Teteris, NJ, Botschner, AW, and McDaniels, B: Traction and compression forces exerted by obstetric forceps and their effect on foetal heart rate. Am J Obst & Gynec 85:1066, 1963.

Wallace, RL, Schifrin, BS, and Paul, RH: The delivery route for very-low-birth-weight infants. Jour Reprod Med 29:736–740, 1984.

Wexler, CA and Burnhill, MS: Method for eliminating difficult mid forceps rotations: Reappraisal of Leff forceps. Am J Obst & Gynec 106:3–9, 1970.

Wylie, B: Forceps traction: An index of birth difficulty. Am J Obst & Gynec 86:38–42, 1963.

Index

A page number in *italics* indicates a figure. A "t" following a page number indicates a table.